fitness
Fast Track to a Better Body

ALL-TIME BEST WORKOUTS TO TONE AND TRIM IN 15 MINUTES

By Betty S. Wong and the Editors of **fitness**

WILEY

John Wiley & Sons, Inc.

This book is printed on acid-free paper. ∞

Copyright © 2011 by Meredith Corporation, Des Moines, Iowa. All rights reserved

Published by John Wiley & Sons, Inc., Hoboken, New Jersey
Published simultaneously in Canada

WRITERS/EDITORS Betty S. Wong, Pamela G. O'Brien, Julia Savacool, Mary Christ Anderson, Bethany Gumper, Sara Wells, Eleanor Langston, Lindsey Emery, Ayren Jackson-Cannady

BOOK DESIGN BY Nichole D'Auria

CONTRIBUTING PHOTO EDITOR Tara Canova

PHOTOGRAPHY BY Peter Ardito: 40, 41, 42, 43; Reggie Casagrande: 133; Denise Crew: 10, 16, 19, 23, 31, 46, 86–87, 104, 110–111, 161, 186, 233; Joey Deleo: 154, 155, 156, 159; Laura Doss: 4–5, 6, 24, 26, 32–33, 38, 53, 109, 112, 134–135, 136, 152, 210, 224; Chris Fanning: 149, 173, 176, 198; Thomas Hoffgen: 164; Sara Kehole: 3, 13, 21, 83, 85, 88, 130, 183, 184–185, 203, 205; Jody Kivort: 147; Erica McConnell: 58–59, 68, 129, 208–209; Alexa Miller: 60; Andrew Parsons: 200; Karen Pearson: 65, 70–77, 96, 97, 99, 101, 103, 116, 120, 121, 122, 124, 141, 143, 144, 150, 151, 169, 171, 172, 175, 178, 179, 192, 194, 195, 197, 199, 201; Amy Postle: 34, 57, 162–163, 181, 207; Melissa Punch: 45; Jay Sullivan: 92–95, 98, 100, 102, 117, 118, 119, 123, 125, 126, 127, 140, 142, 145, 146, 148, 168, 170, 174, 177, 190, 191, 193, 196; David Tsay: 78, 80.

For general information about our other products and services, please contact our Customer Care Department within the United States at (800) 762-2974, outside the United States at (317) 572-3993 or fax (317) 572-4002.

Wiley also publishes its books in a variety of electronic formats. Some content that appears in print may not be available in electronic books. For more information about Wiley products, visit our web site at www.wiley.com.

ISBN 978-0-470-90369-8 (pbk.); ISBN 978-1-118-00839-3 (ebk);
ISBN 978-1-118- 00840-9 (ebk); ISBN 978-1-118- 00841-6 (ebk)

Printed in the United States of America

10 9 8 7 6 5 4 3 2 1

contents

acknowledgments

Creating this book was something like taking a great boot camp class. We pushed ourselves to bring our A game and sweat the details, and once the soreness wore off, we were proud to show off the results. Thanks first and foremost to Mary Anderson, our deputy editor and the head of our fitness department, for her months-long dedication to bringing every page of this book to life. Thanks also to the teamwork of my editors—Pam O'Brien, Julia Savacool, Eleanor Langston, Bethany Gumper, Sara Wells—and FITNESS alums Lindsey Emery and Ayren Jackson-Cannady, even the science within reads as snappy as spandex. Deputy photo editor Tara Canova helped pull together the inspiring images. And making it all look easy was associate art director Nichole D'Auria who designed this book from cover to cover in the most inviting and user-friendly way. Along with their efforts, I want to thank my entire staff for making FITNESS the best magazine in the biz. And to our 7.3 million readers, thank you for being our workout buddies. You're the reason we lace up every morning.

Your Best Body Starts Here

No time? No problem. This book shows you how to slim, strengthen and stick with it—it's easy with our best 15-minute plans.

Busy. It's how most of us would describe our day, our jobs, our lives. When a friend I haven't chatted with in weeks asks "How are you?" my reply is almost automatic: "Oh, good. Busy." I wish it weren't that way, that I could say I woke up this morning to the sounds of birds chirping and then headed outside for a refreshing jog around my neighborhood before getting my two kids off to school and myself to the office. Instead, my morning typically starts with a blaring alarm and ends with my breakfast uneaten, makeup unfinished, and workout undone as I make a mad dash out the door.

Don't worry if this scenario sounds all too familiar. As the editor in chief of FITNESS, I often hear from our readers how hard it is to find time to exercise. But just because you miss an opportunity to work out doesn't mean you can't squeeze in a good sweat session later. Thankfully, choosing to be healthy and fit isn't an all-or-nothing proposition. If I don't get the chance to exercise in the morning, I don't beat myself up over it, because I know the day is still young. Getting your heart rate up and your muscles firing for even as little as 15 minutes a day is enough to make a real difference in your body. We all have 15 minutes—the time it takes for you to watch half of your favorite sitcom, let your manicure dry, or catch up on your friends' latest status updates on Facebook.

We get that you're busy. That's why for nearly 20 years, FITNESS has been serving up the best multitasking moves that tone your entire body. Our reader-favorite column, Express Workout, is the place in the magazine millions of readers love to flip to first to get a fresh routine that will help them firm up, blast fat and get strong—in as little as 15 minutes! We at FITNESS love it, too, challenging the experts we interview each month to reveal their most effective, efficient and fun workout moves and healthy strategies.

My team of editors have gathered so many great ideas—and tried hundreds of kick-butt, hurts-so-good exercises to develop and produce the Express Workout column and our many other exercise features—that we knew we had to share the best of them with you in this book. It's amazing what you can achieve for both your muscles and your mind in just 15 minutes. Whether you want sculpted arms, a sleek back, flat abs, a bootylicious butt or lean legs, we've put together the quick, surefire routines that will help you reach your better-body goal.

Consistency is key, and with all our workouts portioned into 15-minute sessions, who wouldn't find the time to devote to improving her health and body? Once you start seeing results (trust us, you will) and feeling the endorphin boost that exercise delivers, it's easy to stay motivated and positive about fitness. Find the body part you want to concentrate on in the chapters that follow and perform the series of moves shown. Or create your own program based on a combination of moves, like the mixes we've designed in Chapter 9, to keep your body guessing and your muscles continuously challenged. The great thing is that none of our exercises require any fancy or pricey equipment. Just grab a set of dumbbells—if you're a beginner, start with a pair of three- to five-pound weights—and move up to heavier dumbbells as you get stronger. A stability ball, yoga mat and sturdy chair make up the rest of your home gym needs.

Plus, we've packed in plenty of smart advice to help you achieve not only a lean, strong body but also a healthy mind and spirit. After all, exercise is nature's best stress antidote. I know it's the perfect remedy for my frazzled morning and overpacked work schedule.

Especially on days when I miss my morning workout, I'll make a real effort to slip out of the office at lunch and head to the gym for a run on the treadmill or a strength-training session. After a good sweat, I return to work feeling more focused, confident and energized. That's how all the editors at FITNESS get through their busy lives. We work hard but sweat hard, too.

It's easy to sneak in exercise when you appreciate all the good you're doing for your body and life. Whether you squeeze in your workout right when you wake up, in between meetings, before a date or dinner with the family or while you're winding down in front of the TV, 15 minutes is a small pocket of time you can easily find to help you achieve big success. Turn the page to start reaping the muscle and mental rewards of a fit, active lifestyle. *FITNESS Fast Track to a Better Body* is your road map to get moving and get happy in just 15 minutes a day.

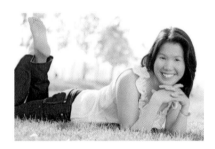

Betty

Betty S. Wong
Editor in Chief of FITNESS

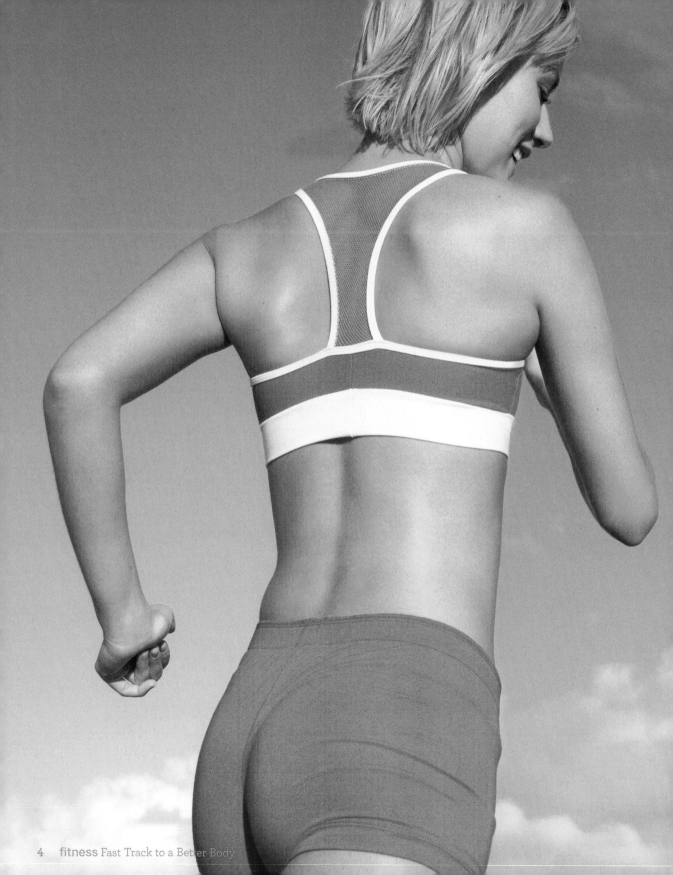

CHAPTER 1

melt more fat

MAXIMIZE YOUR CALORIE BURN DURING EXERCISE AND BEYOND. THESE EASY ADJUSTMENTS HELP YOU GET THE MOST OUT OF EVERY WORKOUT.

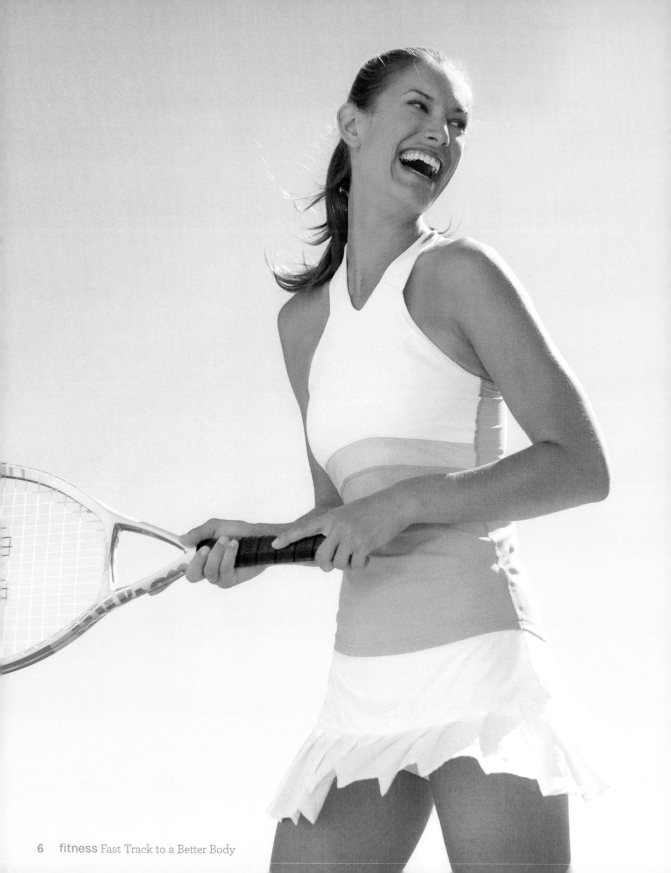

Let's get this straight. The 15-minute workouts in this book will change your shape. Whether you choose to perfect a specific body part from Chapters 4 through 8 or prefer to use those 50 super-effective sculpters à la carte, a regular toning routine will help you achieve a sleeker physique. That's because firming up as you slim down is the fastest way to see wow-body results. Period.

But what about the cardio half of the exercise equation?

You've heard it before: Weight loss is a tug-of-war between calories in, calories out. And the million-dollar question is, Exactly how much exercise does it take to win at that game? Headlines have blared numbers ranging from 10-minute bursts to 90 minutes a day, and the truth is, the right dose is dependent on several key factors.

Cardio exercise is any activity that keeps your heart rate revved up, whether it's mowing the lawn, plugging away on the elliptical trainer or playing a game of tennis. The latest good-for-you guidelines from the American College of Sports Medicine and the American Heart Association call for a minimum of 30 minutes of moderate cardio—think walking at 3 miles per hour—five days a week. Bump up your intensity to the vigorous exercise zone (such as a 4.5-mile-per-hour power walk or a jog) and in that case, say experts, you need just 20 minutes three times a week to get your recommended dose of fitness. You can hit any day's cardio quota either

....

Did You Know?
SWITCHING UP YOUR CARDIO SESSIONS BETWEEN STEADY-PACED WORKOUTS AND INTERVALS IS SMART. "AS WITH A CAR, YOU DON'T ALWAYS WANT TO GUN THE ENGINE," SAYS JOE MASIELLO, CO-OWNER OF FOCUS INTEGRATED FITNESS IN NEW YORK CITY. "INTERVALS ARE GREAT FOR BURNING TONS OF CALORIES, BUT YOUR BODY ALSO NEEDS A DOSE OF LESS INTENSE AEROBICS."

with one continuous workout session or add up 10-minute chunks of activity—your pick.

The reward is a stronger heart and better overall health, no matter which speed you choose. A recent study from the Harvard School of Public Health reveals that exercising at a moderate pace reaps nearly the same cardiovascular disease-reducing benefits as working out at a higher intensity. "As long as you expend equivalent calories, whether you do it at moderate or vigorous intensity does not have much of an impact on disease risk," says Dr. Andrea Chomistek, coauthor of the study.

A quick cue for determining which cardio zone you're in: At a moderate intensity, you should still be able to talk in sentences; at vigorous intensity, you can only get a few words out at a time. Find your zone the next time you set out for a stroll or hit the gym. "Start out at a comfortable pace on the treadmill and increase your speed by .5 mph every 2 minutes, while continuously reciting *The Pledge of Allegiance* out loud," says John Porcari, Ph.D., a FITNESS advisory board member and professor of exercise and sports science at the University of Wisconsin-La Crosse. "When you have to start taking a breath in between every four or five words, that's when you've crossed into vigorous exercise. Reduce your speed to the previous level if you want to stay at your moderate-intensity pace."

Burn Fat Faster

If 20 minutes of cardio three times a week sounds like too little to really make a dent in your weight, you're right. Your heart will benefit, but to shed pounds takes a little more time in your Lycra tights.

How much time depends on your diet. It would be nice if going for a run could erase the ice cream you ate. The truth is, it comes down to how long and fast you run and if you ate the whole pint. Surprised? You're not the only one. Research shows that many women overestimate the number of calories they're blasting daily, sometimes by nearly 1,000!

Q: **WHAT IF I CAN'T GET IN A WORKOUT TODAY?**

A: Don't just sit there when you're stuck at work. Lean people rack up more than two and a half hours of additional daily movement than their overweight peers, a study at the Mayo Clinic in Rochester, Minnesota found. That means they can zap up to 350 extra calories a day on top of their daily exercise. "The calories we burn puttering around are far more important for weight maintenance than we ever imagined," says study author and professor of medicine James Levine, M.D., Ph.D.

Here are the basics: The calories you don't use go straight into reserves (located in Bun 1 and Bun 2, your belly, your hips and your thighs). For every 3,500 calories you torch above and beyond your usual weekly intake, you slim down by about one pound. (More on that in the next chapter.)

As you sit there reading, you're burning about one calorie per minute. That number increases each time you stand, walk or run to grab the phone, because your body needs more energy to get the job done. Scientists measure exercise intensity in METs (metabolic equivalents). The harder you work, the higher your METs. "For weight-loss and health benefits, you should do activities of at least three METs an hour—enough to burn about 200 calories an hour —most days of the week," says Barbara Ainsworth, Ph.D., a professor of exercise and wellness at Arizona State University in Tempe, who helped develop the *Compendium of Physical Activity*, a calorie-burn database.

A recent Harvard University study that sought to finally settle just how much exercise it takes to fend off weight gain pegged that amount at an hour a day. But here's the fine print: Scientists found that the secret to staying slim for the 30,000-plus women they followed was more about calories burned, not time clocked.

The women who successfully maintained a healthy weight completed a total of weekly exercise that was equivalent to 21.5 METs. To reach that magic number, you could do a 3.3-MET activity, like

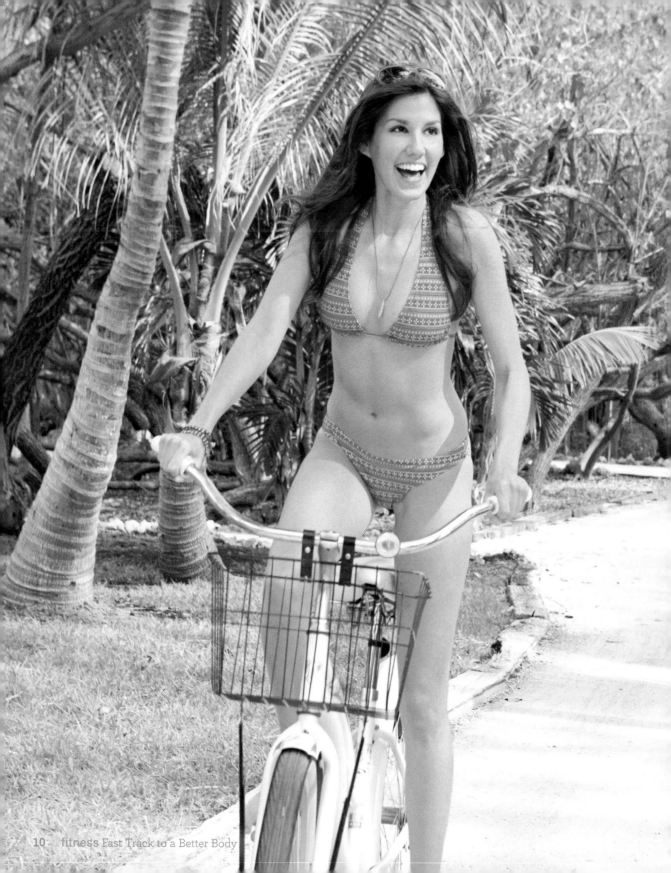

walking at a 20-minute-mile pace, about seven hours a week, or a 10-MET activity, like running at a 10-minute-mile pace, about two hours a week. In other words, do a tougher workout that has a higher MET value and you'll need fewer hours a week to melt enough calories (around 1,300, based on a 140-pound woman) to save your size.

Find your favorite cardio on the chart below and enter its MET value into this formula to see how much weekly exercise time it takes to watch your weight:

21.5 / _____ METs = _____ hours of exercise per week

Exercise Intensity Guide

ACTIVITY		METs
Bicycling (moderate)	>	8
Calisthenics	>	3.5
Circuit Training (cardio intervals)	>	8
Climbing Stairs	>	9
Dancing (general)	>	6.5
Elliptical Trainer (moderate)	>	6.5
Hiking	>	6
In-line Skating	>	12
Jumping Rope	>	10
Pilates	>	3
Running (5 mph)	>	8
Running (6 mph)	>	10
Running (7.5 mph)	>	12.5
Spinning (moderate)	>	7
Swimming (general)	>	6
Walking (3 mph)	>	3.3

But you don't need to memorize that chart to gauge your METs. As a general rule, your MET intensity rises as you:

Move your muscles faster. Your lean tissue is your engine; the more you use, the more fuel you burn.

Pull your own weight. Activities you do while standing up, like running, burn more calories at a higher level than those in which your weight is supported, such as cycling. The trade-off: You can usually do the sit-down activity longer to make up the difference.

Work harder. Walking uphill uses more energy than level strolling. Cranking the knob on a stationary bike ups your burn.

To see how your favorite activities convert to calories burned per hour, check out these at-a-glance groupings of some of the most popular workout choices. Aim to burn at least 300 calories per session if you're exercising for weight loss, suggest experts.

Big Burners
400 to 500+ calories per hour

ACTIVITY		BURNS
Elliptical Training	>	575
Mountain Biking	>	545
Circuit Training (hard, with some cardio between sets)	>	510
Cross-Country Skiing (moderate)	>	510
Rowing (moderate, stationary machine)	>	450
Swimming (free-style laps, easy)	>	450

Steady Scorchers
300 to 400+ calories per hour

ACTIVITY		BURNS
Weight Lifting (dumbbells or machines)	>	385
Hiking (without a pack)	>	385
Walk-Jog Intervals	>	350
Body-Sculpting Class	>	510
Kayaking	>	450
Jazz Dance	>	450
Power Walking (very briskly, 4 mph)	>	320

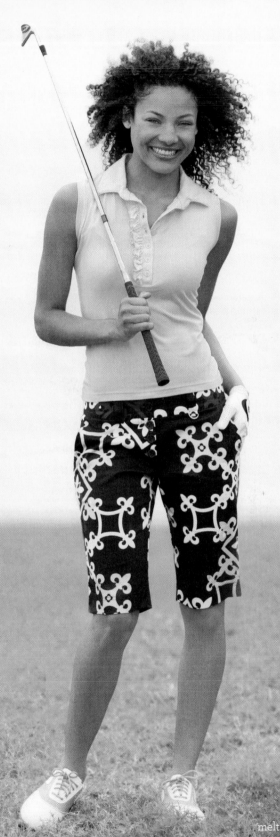

Easy Slimmers
150 to 300+ calories per hour

ACTIVITY		BURNS
Flamenco, Belly or Swing Dancing	>	290
Shooting Hoops	>	290
Golfing (walking and carrying clubs)	>	290
Water Aerobics	>	255
Tai Chi	>	255
Brisk Walking (3.5 mph)	>	245
Pilates (general mat workout)	>	160
Yoga (hatha)	>	160

The M Factor

The key to burning more calories 24/7

Metabolism sounds mysterious and complicated, but it's actually pretty simple: It's the amount of energy (aka calories) our bodies need daily, for everything from breathing to eating to exercising, says Rochelle Goldsmith, Ph.D., director of the Exercise Physiology Lab at Columbia University Medical Center in New York City. The trouble begins when you consume more calories than your body needs to do these things. That's when you start to pack on the pounds.

You can partly thank your parents for the speed of your metabolism, or the rate with which your body consumes fuel for these activities. Genes contribute to the levels of appetite-control hormones we have floating around in our bodies, Goldsmith explains. "Some people are genetically programmed to be active; they're naturally restless and use more energy," she says. Gender also plays a role. "The average man's metabolism is about 10 to 15 percent higher than a woman's," Goldsmith notes. That's mainly because men have more muscle mass than women do, which means they burn more calories. "Muscle does the work to help you move, while fat just sits there," says physiologist John Porcari, Ph.D. Not only that, but women's bodies are designed to hold on to body fat in case of pregnancy.

Crank Up Your Metabolism

The good news is, you can make your metabolism faster, experts say, despite genetics and gender. These are the five simple exercise secrets to boosting yours.

Did You Know?
THE BREATHING, BLINKING AND THINKING YOU DO EACH DAY USE UP ABOUT 70 PERCENT OF YOUR TOTAL DAILY CALORIES. TO TALLY UP THE CALORIC BURN OF YOUR SO-CALLED BASAL METABOLIC RATE, DIVIDE YOUR WEIGHT BY 2.2, THEN MULTIPLY BY 24.

1. Exercise more often. Working out is the number-one way to keep your furnace stoked by helping you build more lean muscle. Exercise enough and you can help prevent the natural metabolic slowdown that begins as early as your late twenties.

Your amp-it-up plan: five workouts a week. "Do three days of aerobic activity and two days of weight lifting," advises Shawn Talbott, Ph.D., an exercise physiologist, a nutritional biochemist and the executive producer of *Killer at Large,* a documentary about the U.S. obesity epidemic.

2. Kick up your cardio. Aerobic intervals keep your metabolic rate higher than a steady-pace routine does for as long as an hour after you stop exercising, according to FITNESS advisory board member Michele Olson, Ph.D., professor of exercise science at Auburn University at Montgomery in Alabama. A basic metabolism-boosting interval routine is to "go hard for a couple of minutes, then take it down to an easier pace for a minute or two, and keep alternating like that throughout your workout," Talbott says. (Flip to Workouts That Keep on Working on page 22 for more easy-to-follow interval plans.)

Just pick your cardio wisely. Aim for exercises that require your body to work its hardest by using multiple muscle groups, Talbott says. That means hitting kickboxing class is better than riding a stationary bike. Or try a circuit of cardio exercises. "Do a variety of activities—like running stadium stairs, jumping rope and squat thrusts—for two minutes each, aiming for a total of 10 minutes," Olson says. "That will really rock your metabolism."

3. Put some muscle behind it. Too many women steer clear of strength training, fearing that they'll bulk up. Don't make this mistake. A head-to-toe strength routine will turbocharge your calorie-blasting quotient. Add five pounds of muscle to your body and you can zap as many as 600 calories an hour during your usual

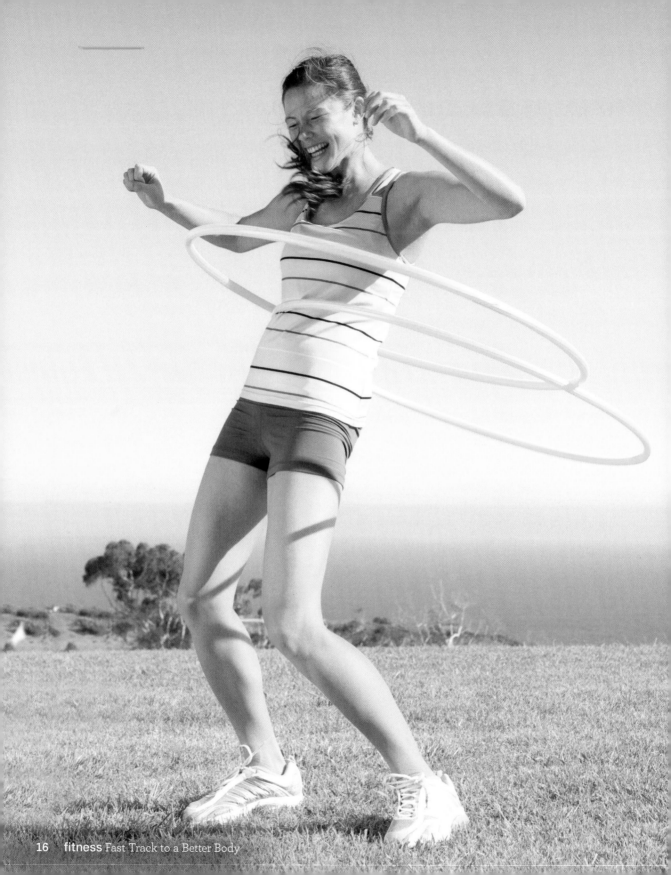

workout, Olson says. Be sure to choose a weight-lifting routine that targets your core, legs, arms, chest and shoulders; challenging numerous muscles will help your body function like a calorie-burning machine, according to Goldsmith. (Find some great total-body strength workouts in Chapter 9.)

4. Get off your butt. Sitting too much—at the computer at work, at home in front of the TV—slows your metabolism, even if you're exercising regularly. An easy fix is to stretch, stroll and fidget throughout the day. That's what scientists call NEAT, or nonexercise activity thermogenesis, and it can boost your burn and help you drop weight, says medical professor James Levine, M.D., Ph.D. The proof: In a study of lean volunteers who were fed extra calories, those who paced frequently, for example, maintained their weight, while the people who did no additional walking got chubbier. If you take advantage of every opportunity to walk and climb stairs, it can make a big difference. "A woman who needs to lose weight would have to burn about 190 to 200 extra calories a day to lose 10 percent of her body weight, which you can do by increasing your overall activity level," Goldsmith says. "Try striding around your house or office when you're on the phone, standing up at your desk whenever you can and walking to your coworker's cube instead of e-mailing her."

5. Schedule a nighttime workout. Do a 20- to 30-minute moderate-intensity cardio routine before you hit the hay to keep your metabolism humming all night, Porcari says. The average woman's metabolic rate naturally decreases by about 15 percent while she sleeps, but an end-of-day sweat session will make the drop closer to 5 percent, he explains. Take the dog for an evening walk or go for a bike ride with your family after dinner. And don't worry that the activity will keep you awake: As long as you exercise at least two and a half hours before going to bed, you should be able to drift off with no problem, experts say.

5 Common Calorie Myths Busted

Get off the treadmill to nowhere by exercising smarter.

Myth: Mile per mile, running and walking burn the same.
The real deal: Not even close. "Running is a more energetic activity, because you're jumping off the ground with each stride," says David Swain, Ph.D., a professor of exercise science and director of the Wellness Institute and Research Center at Old Dominion University in Norfolk, Virginia. Per mile, running burns about twice as many calories.

Myth: You need to stay in the fat-burning zone to slim down.
The real deal: "Because fat takes longer than carbs to be converted to energy, you burn a higher percentage of it when you're walking than when you're running. So the old thinking was that with low-intensity exercise you could torch body fat and lose weight," explains physiologist John Porcari, Ph.D. But the theory didn't work in practice. "In one study, we had people walk or run for half an hour. On average, the walkers burned 240 calories, 44 percent of which were fat, so they burned 108 fat calories. The runners burned 450 calories, 24 percent of which were fat, so they burned 120 fat calories. Whether you look at total calories or fat calories, the runners clearly came out ahead," Porcari says. The solution: There's nothing wrong with low-intensity exercise—particularly if you have joint problems—but to lose weight, you'll likely need to do it for longer than half an hour.

Myth: You can't trust those numbers on the treadmill.
The real deal: Years ago, the calorie-burn indicators on some

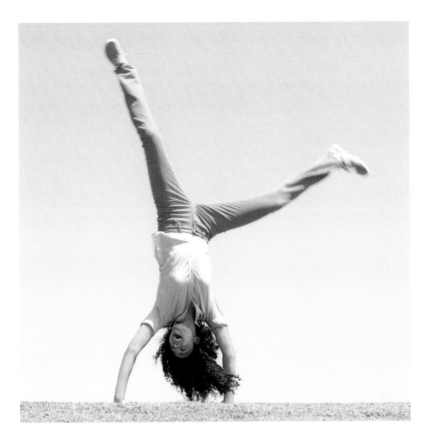

popular gym machines were reported to be notoriously inaccurate. "These days, they do a pretty good job," says metabolism researcher Gary Hunter, Ph.D., of the University of Alabama at Birmingham, "especially if you program in your weight."

Myth: You burn more in the cold.
The real deal: It's true that you incinerate calories when you're shivering. But once you warm up during your workout, you won't use more energy than usual just because it's chilly outside.

Myth: High-calorie-burning exercises are best.
The real deal: "For many women, what burns the most is the activity they can sustain for a long time, like power walking or hiking," says Arizona State University professor of exercise and wellness Barbara Ainsworth, Ph.D.

Walk It Off

Yes! You can lose weight with this simple stride guide.

Check out the latest skinny on walking: Women between the ages of 18 and 30 who walked at least four hours a week were 44 percent more likely to lose weight during the 15 years they were tracked than those who didn't walk at all—regardless of what other exercise they did, according to a study in the *American Journal of Clinical Nutrition*. For maximum results, keep your pace at three miles per hour or peppier as you aim to hit that 240-minute-a-week total. Alternate in these three walks to your usual routine for an added body boost.

Walk 1: Hills

Tackling hills or stairs will sculpt your legs and butt while burning big calories—58 percent more at a 17-minute-mile pace.

- Start out on a flat surface for 15 minutes at a speed at which you're hustling but still able to speak in sentences (your rate of perceived exertion, or RPE, on a scale of 1 to 10, where 1 is sitting still and 10 is a full-tilt sprint, should be about 6 or 7).

- Find a hill or some steps—or set your treadmill to a 4 to 6 percent incline—and walk uphill quickly for 2 minutes.

- Walk downhill to recover, or if you're on a treadmill, walk at a 0 percent incline for 2 minutes.

- Maintain pace or go faster so that you can speak just a few words at a time (RPE: 8). Only one set of stairs? Walk up and down for 4 minutes.

- Continue up- and downhill walking intervals until you've reached your time goal. Beginners can alternate between hills and 5 minutes on a flat surface.

CALORIES BURNED (45 MINUTES):
220 (17-minute mile) to 366 (13-minute mile)

Did You Know? TO BURN MORE CALORIES EVERY DAY, MIND YOUR STEP! SIMPLY JOTTING DOWN YOUR WALKING MILEAGE COULD SPUR YOU TO GO AN EXTRA QUARTER MILE OR MORE DAILY, FINDS A STUDY OF PEDOMETER USERS AT LOUGHBOROUGH UNIVERSITY IN LEICESTERSHIRE, ENGLAND.

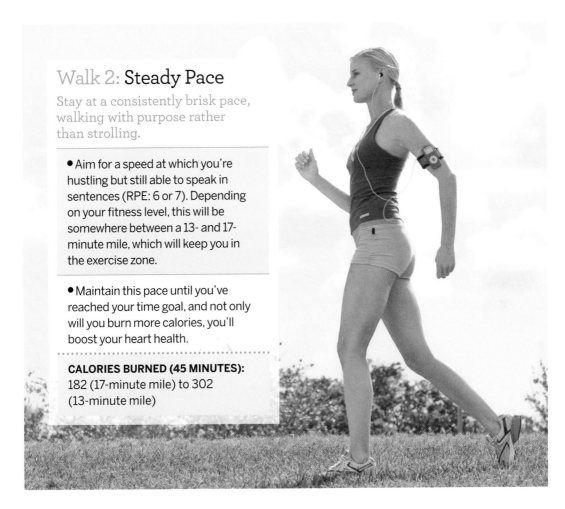

Walk 2: Steady Pace

Stay at a consistently brisk pace, walking with purpose rather than strolling.

- Aim for a speed at which you're hustling but still able to speak in sentences (RPE: 6 or 7). Depending on your fitness level, this will be somewhere between a 13- and 17-minute mile, which will keep you in the exercise zone.

- Maintain this pace until you've reached your time goal, and not only will you burn more calories, you'll boost your heart health.

CALORIES BURNED (45 MINUTES):
182 (17-minute mile) to 302
(13-minute mile)

Walk 3: Intervals

You'll torch more fat in less time by increasing your pace a little—accelerating from a 17-minute mile to a 13-minute mile, for instance, means you'll burn 66 percent more calories.

- Warm up at your regular pace (RPE: 6) for 6 minutes.

- Alternate these intervals: Walk as fast as you can for 1 minute (RPE: 8), then slow down to your regular pace (RPE: 6) for 2 minutes to recover.

- Repeat intervals until you've reached your time goal.

CALORIES BURNED (45 MINUTES):
241 (17-minute mile) to 326 (13-minute mile)

Workouts That Keep On Working

If you are ready to get sweaty, try one of these three fat-blasting interval sessions guaranteed to give you a bigger afterburn.

The harder you exercise, the longer your body continues to zap calories even after you've toweled off. "Both types of cardio workouts—moderate and vigorous—have their benefits," says physiologist Michele Olson, Ph.D. "But you'll see more physical changes by picking up the intensity every now and then."

Why? "High-intensity exercise increases the release of growth hormones, which mobilize fat to be used as fuel, plus it causes your metabolism to stay elevated about 10 to 15 percent above its baseline post-workout," says Arthur Weltman, Ph.D., director of the Exercise Physiology Laboratory at the University of Virginia in Charlottesville. In other words, if you worked off 300 calories during your session, you'll get a bonus burn of about 45 calories even after you've toweled off. In fact, studies show you can net nine times the fat loss by doing intervals rather than keeping a steady pace.

To get the effect, infuse your favorite cardio routine—walking, running, biking, swimming, elliptical trainer, etc.—with the high-energy intervals given on the following pages to boost your afterburn by up to 100 calories. The best part? We've made these interval sequences simple to remember, even without the cheat sheets, so you can concentrate on your workout and not your number-crunching skills!

Did You Know? INTERVALS ARE HIGHLY STRESSFUL ON YOUR BODY, SO TO PREVENT INJURY, EACH HIGH-INTENSITY DAY SHOULD BE FOLLOWED BY AT LEAST ONE OR TWO DAYS OF REST OR LIGHT ACTIVITY, LIKE WALKING OR CYCLING.

The Countdown

Total time: 35 minutes

Do the speed bursts here at the fastest pace you can safely maintain (power walking, running, cycling, using the elliptical or stairclimber) for the given duration. Then blast off with short, all-out sprints.

Warm up for 5 minutes.

SPEED BURST		EASY-PACE RECOVERY
4 minutes	❭	4 minutes
3 minutes	❭	3 minutes
2 minutes	❭	2 minutes
1 minute	❭	1 minute

Blast off!

SPEED BURST		EASY-PACE RECOVERY
30 seconds	❭	1 minute
30 seconds	❭	1 minute
30 seconds	❭	1 minute
30 seconds	❭	1 minute

Cool down for 4 minutes.

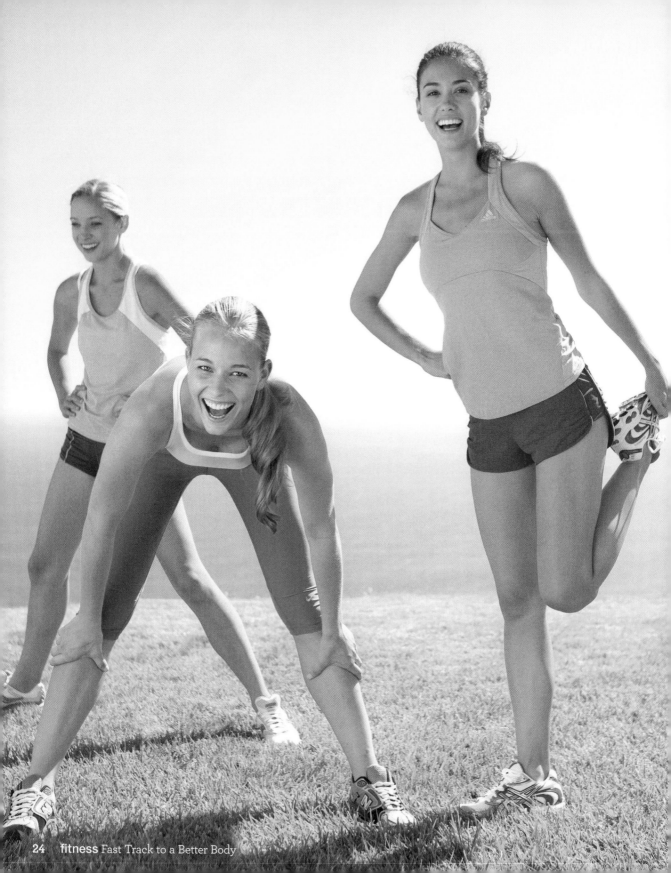

The Quickie

Total time: 16 (advanced) to 29 (beginner) minutes

It's easy: Speed up for the number of seconds listed for your level, then go at an easy pace for a minute or two to recover. Repeat 8 times for a complete cardio session.

Warm up for 5 minutes:

- 3 minutes light walk or jog ● 30 seconds at half effort ● 30 seconds light walk or jog ● 30 seconds at 75 percent of maximum effort ● 30 seconds light walk or jog

CHOOSE ONE OF THE LEVELS BELOW AND REPEAT 8 TIMES TO COMPLETE YOUR SESSION.

LEVEL		SPRINT		RECOVERY
Beginner	❯	60-second jog	❯	20-second walk
Intermediate	❯	30-second sprint	❯	60-to-90-second walk
Advanced	❯	20-second sprint	❯	60-second walk

The Reverse

Total time: 34 minutes

Start out faster than normal (power walk, run, cycle, use the elliptical or stairclimber at a challenging level) and slow down every 3 minutes until you hit an easy pace. The intensity levels listed are on a scale of 1 to 10, where 1 is lounging and 10 is an all-out sprint; an 8.5, for example, is 85 percent of your maximum effort. The key is to find your starting speed. If you start out too fast and get fatigued, slow down to recover, then pick up where you left off when ready.

Warm up for 5 minutes.

INTENSITY LEVEL (on a scale of 1 to 10)		TIME
8.5	❯	3 minutes
8	❯	3 minutes
7.5	❯	3 minutes
7	❯	3 minutes
6.5	❯	3 minutes
6	❯	3 minutes
5.5	❯	3 minutes
5	❯	3 minutes

Cool down for 5 minutes.

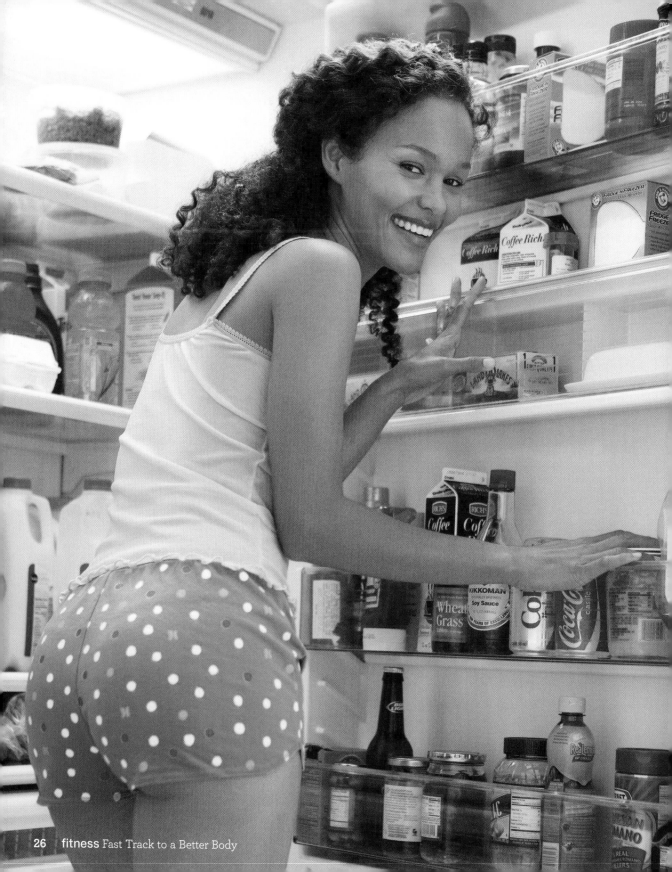

Nix Post-Workout Pig-Outs

Ways to find willpower when you need it most

If you believe a hotly contested idea currently being circulated among researchers and making big headlines, exercise, ironically, is being singled out in some circles as a deterrent to weight loss efforts. "There's this hunger issue," admits Kendrin Sonneville, R.D., a researcher at Harvard School of Public Health whose study found that kids who exercised the most ate back all the calories they burned off, and then some. Could exercise really be a big waste of time? Sonneville's reply: "No, but it's not a panacea for weight loss either, because exercise increases your appetite. The food/exercise equation is imbalanced. It may take an hour to burn 500 calories, but only five minutes to eat them."

And that's exactly what your body wants you to do. "In the short term, during or right after a workout, exercise may suppress hunger," says Barry Braun, Ph.D., director of the Energy Metabolism Laboratory at the University of Massachusetts in Amherst. "But later that day or the next day, your hunger hormones can surge, making you want to eat. At the same time, your body's satiety hormones—the ones that signal to you that you're full—may decrease." The really unfair part, Braun notes, is that the desire to eat more after exercising hits women harder than men. "When we look at blood samples of men and women starting an exercise program, there's a subtle change in men's hormone levels, but for women, exercise really elevates the hormone that increases your appetite," he says. "The widely accepted theory is that women's bodies are hardwired to hold onto energy for reproduction purposes." So when your body senses that you're burning fuel from exercise, it wants to make sure you replace it pronto.

All of which means that for women who love fitness, and want to be toned as well as trim, shedding pounds poses a unique challenge of balancing calories in, calories out, female hormones and exercise-induced hunger pangs. But the payoff is well worth it: "What all the latest news stories missed is the role exercise plays in keeping the pounds off in the long run," says Timothy Church, M.D., Ph.D., a professor at the Pennington Biomedical Research Center in Baton Rouge, who has done extensive research on the factors that influence successful weight loss. "It's a fact that the only people who keep off the weight they've lost are the ones who are physically active."

Those who use dieting alone to take off pounds usually find themselves right back where they started, or even heavier, studies show. Beyond the scale, exercise offers other major benefits: It blasts dangerous belly fat, reduces your risk of high cholesterol, heart disease and diabetes, and makes you happy, each of which can help you live longer.

Hunger on the Brain

The key to sticking with your workout—and your diet—while dodging the stomach rumbling and constant cravings is to understand the relationship between energy (food) and exercise, and learn to use both to your advantage. The first step is decoding where the hunger is coming from.

Happy hunger: Finishing a tough workout makes you feel proud. So proud you'd like to celebrate your hard work—preferably with a large vanilla cone and rainbow sprinkles! "I have so many clients who have this perception that if they work out they can reward themselves by eating whatever they want and they'll still lose weight," says Dawn Jackson Blatner, R.D., a FITNESS advisory board member. That kind of thinking can backfire. "To placate hunger while still dropping pounds, I tell clients to eat back no more than half of the calories they burned off during a workout," says Blatner. "So if you burn 300 calories jogging, you have 150 calories to play with during the day." The trick is maximizing your nutritional quality in minimal calories. You could use up those 150 calories with a sugary drink—the wrong move, since liquid calories won't satisfy hunger. "Ideally you'd spend those calories on filling foods, such as a sliced apple with peanut butter, to maximize satiety," says Blatner.

Fear hunger: On the other end of the spectrum, some women are afraid to consume calories before their sweat session, figuring they'll only negate the purpose of 60 minutes on the elliptical. That's a big mistake—working out on an empty stomach means you won't have the energy to exercise as long or as hard, so you'll end up burning fewer overall calories than if you'd amped up your stamina with a 200-calorie pre-workout snack and pushed your way through a tough session, says Leslie Bonci, R.D., director of sports nutrition at the University of Pittsburgh Medical Center and a FITNESS advisory board member. "Eating something, such as a piece of fruit before exercise, may help give you more energy and stamina during your workout," agrees Blatner.

Rebellion hunger: Leaving your fuel supply depleted post-workout is similarly shortsighted. Eventually you will get hungry—really hungry—particularly for fatty food. "When we're starving, we have an innate desire to quickly consume energy-dense food," says Sonneville. So rather than holding off, then scarfing down 600 calories with two mega brownies a couple of hours after your workout, do the smart thing and spend 150 calories right after the gym on a low-fat yogurt.

Little Changes That Add Up

When you're low on motivation, try these four tricks for getting in that sweat session today.

Be an early bird to get the workout. Lace up first thing and you'll increase your odds of exercising threefold. A study of 500 people at the Mollen Clinic, a preventive medicine and wellness center in Scottsdale, Arizona, found that 75 percent of those who worked out in the morning did so regularly, compared with just half the afternoon exercisers and a quarter of the post-work crowd.

Heed the 10-minute rule. Forget the all-or-nothing attitude toward exercise and you may never skip another workout session. "When you're not in the mood to work out, tell yourself that you'll just do 10 minutes," says celebrity trainer Jay Kerwin. "Once you get going, you'll remember why you're there and probably stick it out for a full routine."

Enlist a workout buddy. If you're currently flying solo, recruit a pal who will hold you accountable for those 7 a.m. workouts. Walkers and runners can link up with like-minded striders at rrca.org, cyclists at specializedriders.com and swimmers at clubswim.com.

Liven up your living room. If you miss your fair-weather routine, re-create it indoors. Turn your road bike into a stationary one by mounting it on a bike trainer or keep running without the trail with a mini-trampoline. And bring a touch of the outdoors inside to help you get your nature fix: Open up the shades and put some low-maintenance plants, like bamboo or ferns, in your exercise space.

Did You Know?
TRYING TO WORK OUT AND WORK THROUGH A MENTAL CHALLENGE AT THE SAME TIME SENDS STRESS HORMONE LEVELS THROUGH THE ROOF, WARNS A STUDY FROM MISSISSIPPI STATE UNIVERSITY IN STARKVILLE. LEAVE YOUR MENTAL TO-DO LIST AT HOME DURING SWEAT SESSIONS AND TUNE IN TO YOUR PLAYLIST INSTEAD.

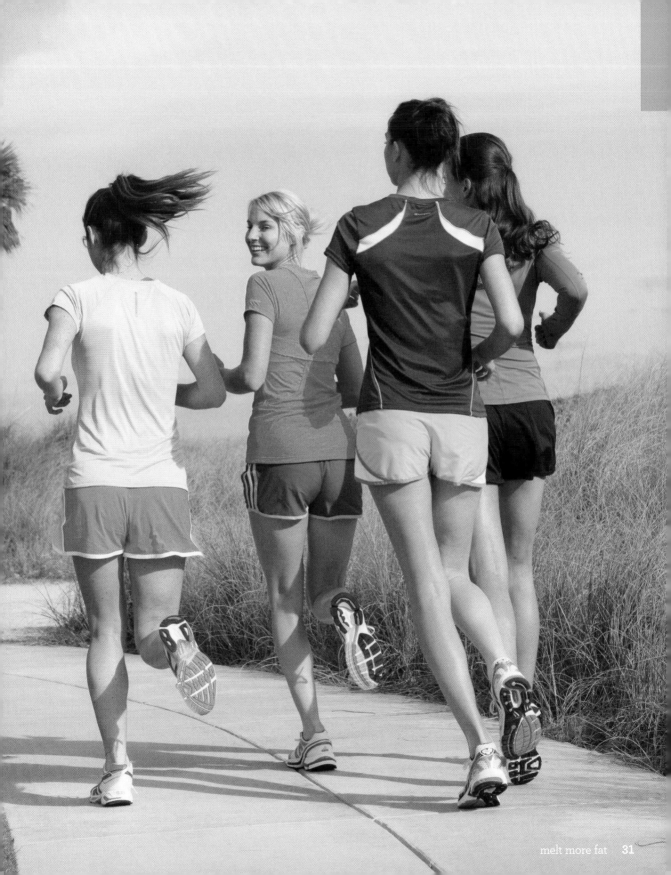

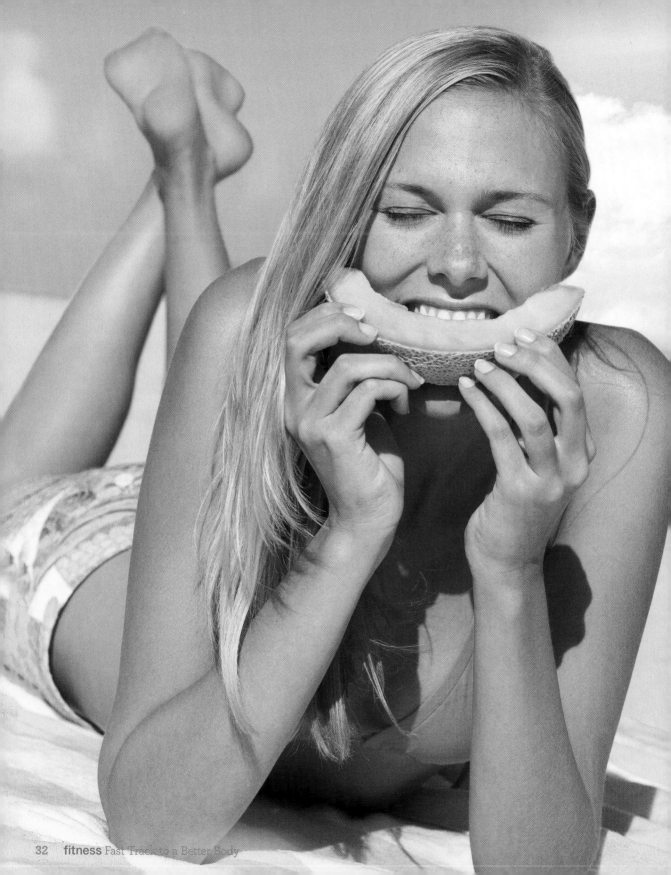

CHAPTER 2

eat
your way
slim

ACHIEVE LASTING WEIGHT LOSS WITH
THIS NO-DEPRIVATION DIET, PLUS
STRATEGIES FOR INCREASING YOUR
METABOLISM AND KICKING CRAVINGS.

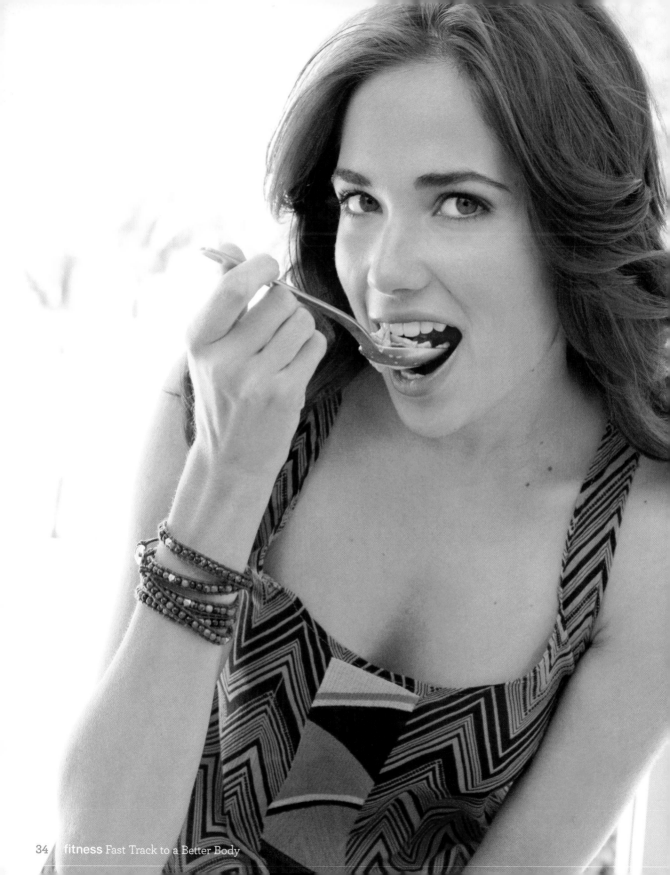

How many times has someone tried to tell you that a certain diet is "easy?" Sure it is, if you (A) have several hours a day to chop fruit, grill chicken and roast vegetables, (B) eat every meal in your own kitchen, (C) dislike chocolate, burgers and pizza, or (D) all of the above.

But the Eat More, Lose More diet on the following pages *is* easy. You'll drop at least five pounds in one month, without spending hours in the kitchen or giving up your favorite foods. The secret: small changes that add up to big results. Starting your day with breakfast. Choosing turkey over tuna salad in your six-inch sub at lunch (do it every day and you'll lose 25 pounds over the next year!). Eating every three hours.

The tasty, 1,500-calorie-a-day menus were designed by the nutrition pros on the FITNESS advisory board to fill you up and fit into your lifestyle. But even before you dig in, it's good to know a few basics for beating the road blocks that have been keeping you from your goal weight.

You run your butt off on the treadmill, you eat healthy (sometimes to the point of a seriously grumbly stomach) and still the pounds won't budge. What's the deal?

Weight loss isn't magic. Remember, one pound equals 3,500 calories. (That's the equivalent of four sticks of butter —yikes!) So to lose one pound you must burn and/or cut a total of 3,500 calories.

· · · · · · · · · · · · · · · · · · · ·

Did You Know?
A UNIVERSITY OF NORTH CAROLINA STUDY FOUND THAT AMERICANS EAT AN AVERAGE OF 115 CALORIES MORE PER DAY ON FRIDAY, SATURDAY AND SUNDAY THAN THEY DO ON WEEKDAYS, WHICH ADDS UP TO AN EXTRA FIVE POUNDS A YEAR.

Look at it another way: To drop that pound in seven days, you would need to reduce your net calories by 500 every day; you could cut 250 calories from your diet and work off 250 more with exercise, for instance. To lose two pounds in a week, you'd have to double your savings to 1,000 calories a day, but don't dip below that—losing anything more than two pounds a week is considered unsafe.

Meanwhile, a girl's best friend in the weight-loss game is her metabolism. In Chapter 1, you learned how exercise can help get yours humming. Taking the right bites can likewise increase the rate at which you burn calories even on days you miss a workout.

Your first step to stacking the fat-melting deck in your favor? Have breakfast. An a.m. meal is key to jump-starting your metabolism first thing; otherwise, it's still running at the same speed it was as you slept. Plus, researchers have shown that people who eat breakfast consume less over the course of the day.

Second, eat often. Seriously: Studies suggest that people who nosh throughout the day are less likely to be heavy. Meal-skipping can slow your metabolism and boost levels of the hunger hormone ghrelin. Too much time between meals puts your insulin levels on a roller coaster (translation: ravenous hunger!). So don't go longer than three hours without a healthy meal or snack.

And finally, no starving yourself! Eating too few calories can backfire because you're more likely to lose metabolism-revving lean muscle, not fat. Don't dip below about 1,100 calories a day.

Outsmart Diet Pitfalls

Think back to your last diet. How long did it last? Research shows that a quarter of dieters fall off the wagon within 14 days. That's why the Eat More, Lose More diet was designed to tackle the three biggest reasons most diets fail.

Diet trap: The all-or-nothing mentality. You swear off all your favorite foods and hit the gym seven days a week. You're so gung-ho

Q: I CAN'T GET THE LAST FIVE POUNDS TO BUDGE. WHAT GIVES?

Q: I CAN'T GET THE LAST FIVE POUNDS TO BUDGE. WHAT GIVES?

A: First, ask yourself whether you've set a goal weight that's too low— your body may be telling you that the weight would be hard to maintain. "If you're sure you need to keep losing, remember that the final five pounds are very different from the first," says weight loss expert Madelyn Fernstrom, Ph.D., author of *The Real You Diet*. The more weight you drop, the fewer calories your body needs—so it becomes harder to create the deficit required to trim down. Aim to shed 2 pounds a month (instead of per week, like you did when you had more to lose) by burning 250 more calories than you consume every day. Here's how: Shave 100 to 150 calories off your daily diet (skip your nightly glass of wine, for example) while you also burn an extra 100 to 150 calories (jog for 10 minutes more or take three 10-minute walks throughout the day).

to slim down that you try to do too much too soon, which causes you to quit.

Sidestep it: On the Eat More, Lose More diet, you make small changes you can stick with for good. The tasty meals help you cut calories on the sly, so you never feel deprived.

Diet trap: The guessing game. You can order grilled cheese instead of grilled chicken, because you ran an extra mile, right? Not so fast. Research shows that many women seriously underestimate the number of calories they eat and overestimate the number they burn.

Sidestep it: On the plan, you'll know exactly what to eat to lose weight, learning proper portion sizes, so you can maintain your weight loss for life.

Diet trap: Cinderella syndrome. Your diet is a fairy-tale fantasy with no room for slipups. As soon as life interferes—a birthday party, dinner out, happy hour—it's all over.

Sidestep it: Included in this chapter are proven stay-motivated secrets to keep you on track. Now, turn the page to get started!

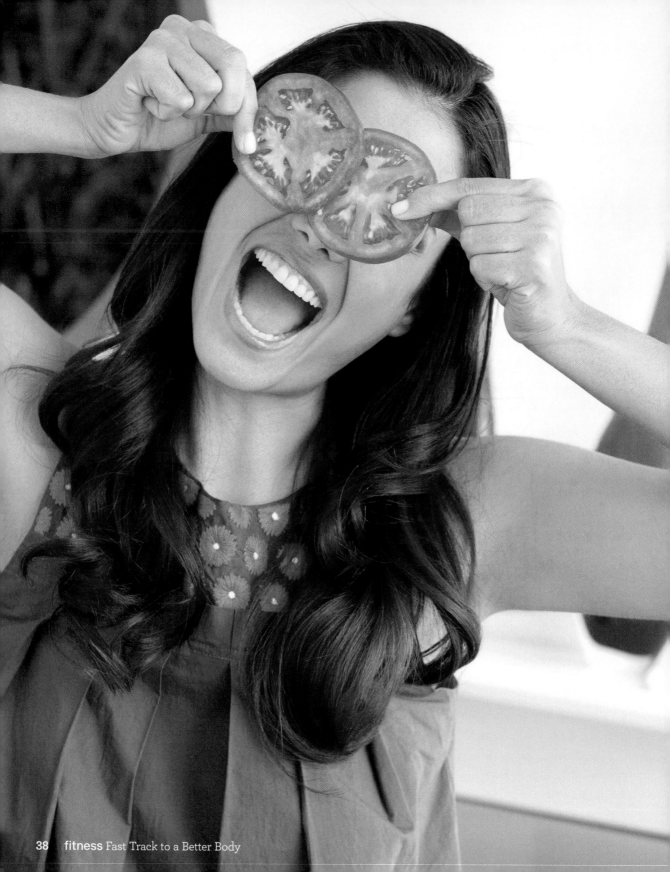

The Eat More, Lose More Diet

Fill up and slim down with these satisfying menus.

This diet food tastes great! We know you've heard that line before, but just take a peek at the delicious recipes you can eat in one day on this plan: cinnamon French toast for breakfast, nachos with black beans for lunch, and a burger with fries for dinner. Still hungry? Snack on chips and dip or popcorn and peanuts.

There are no gimmicks here, just one simple equation: a 300-calorie breakfast + a 400-calorie lunch + a 500-calorie dinner + two 150-calorie snacks = results. These menus were devised by nutrition gurus to make sure you get all the nutrients you need for those calories. The quick, easy meals supply whole grains, lean protein and healthy fats—a winning combination that will keep you satisfied for hours. Choose from the breakfasts, lunches, snacks and dinners on these pages for a total of 1,500 calories a day (remember, no meal-skipping allowed). Because that's 500 less than what the typical woman eats in a day, you'll drop five pounds in one month— add exercise and you'll double that amount.

Portion Control
Get a handle on proper single serving sizes here.

• ½ cup cooked brown rice or spaghetti	❭ ½ baseball
• ⅔ cup cooked oatmeal	❭ 1 tennis ball
• 1 ounce bread	❭ 1 slice the size of a CD case
• 3 ounces cooked salmon or chicken	❭ 1 deck of cards
• 1 ounce nuts	❭ 1 golf ball
• 1 tbsp peanut butter	❭ ½ walnut

Healthy Breakfasts (about 300 calories each)

Maple-Pear French Toast

Add 1 teaspoon butter to a skillet. In a bowl, whisk together 1 egg and 1 egg white. Dip 2 slices whole-wheat cinnamon bread in egg; add bread to pan. Cook 2 minutes per side. Toss ½ pear, sliced, with 1 tablespoon light pancake syrup and spoon over toast.

Tomato and Goat Cheese Frittata

Mist a skillet with nonstick cooking spray. Whisk together 1 egg and 2 egg whites. Add a pinch of salt and pepper; pour into pan. When eggs are halfway set, add 5 halved grape tomatoes and ½ ounce crumbled goat cheese. Cook until fully set, about 5 minutes. Serve with 1 slice whole-grain toast.

Southwestern Breakfast Wrap

Mist a frying pan with nonstick cooking spray. Whisk together 1 egg, 2 egg whites, 2 tablespoons salsa and a pinch of salt and pepper. Pour into pan and scramble. Spoon onto 1 whole-wheat tortilla. Top with 1 tablespoon shredded reduced-fat cheddar cheese, ½ cup chopped tomato, 1 tablespoon chopped cilantro and 2 more tablespoons salsa. Roll up.

Potato Hash and Cheddar Omelet

Mist pan with nonstick cooking spray. Add ½ cup preshredded potatoes and cook for 5 minutes, turning once. Add 1 whole egg plus 2 egg whites, whisked together; 1 cup baby spinach; and salt and pepper to taste. Cook for an additional 4 minutes, or until egg is done and spinach is wilted. Top with 4 tablespoons shredded cheddar cheese.

Cream Cheese and Lox Wrap

Spread 1½ tablespoons low-fat cream cheese on an 8-inch whole-wheat wrap. Top with 3 ounces smoked salmon, 2 slices tomato, 2 slices red onion and a handful of sprouts. Roll up.

Almond and Apple English Muffin

Toast a whole-wheat English muffin. On half, spread 1 tablespoon almond butter and top with ½ apple, thinly sliced, and a sprinkle of cinnamon; cover with the remaining muffin half.

Roasted Apricots Over Greek Yogurt

Preheat oven to 450°. Halve 2 to 3 ripe apricots; place in a glass baking dish, cover with foil and roast 20 minutes. (Apricots can be roasted the night before.) Mix 1 cup nonfat Greek yogurt with 2 tablespoons slivered almonds and a drizzle of honey. Top with apricots.

POTATO HASH AND CHEDDAR OMELET

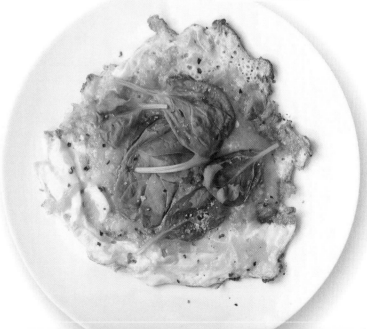

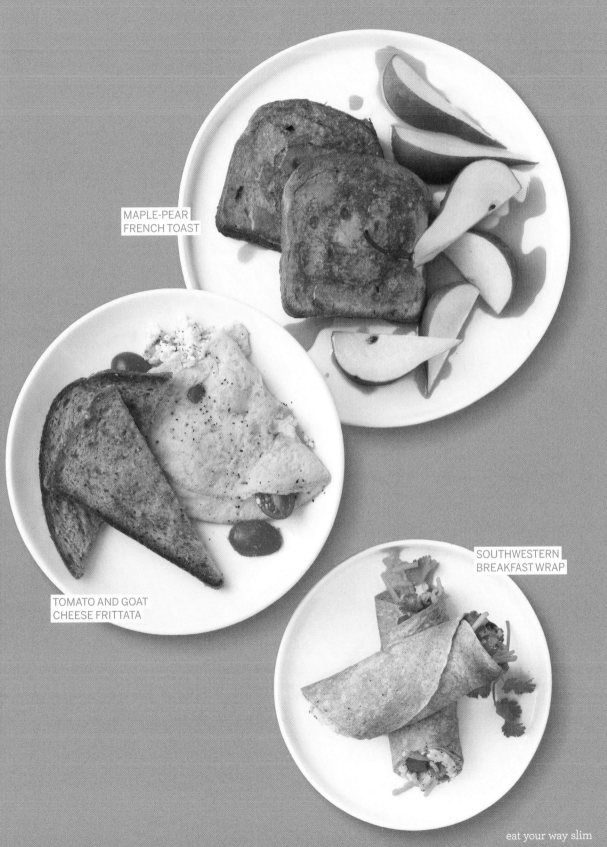

MAPLE-PEAR
FRENCH TOAST

TOMATO AND GOAT
CHEESE FRITTATA

SOUTHWESTERN
BREAKFAST WRAP

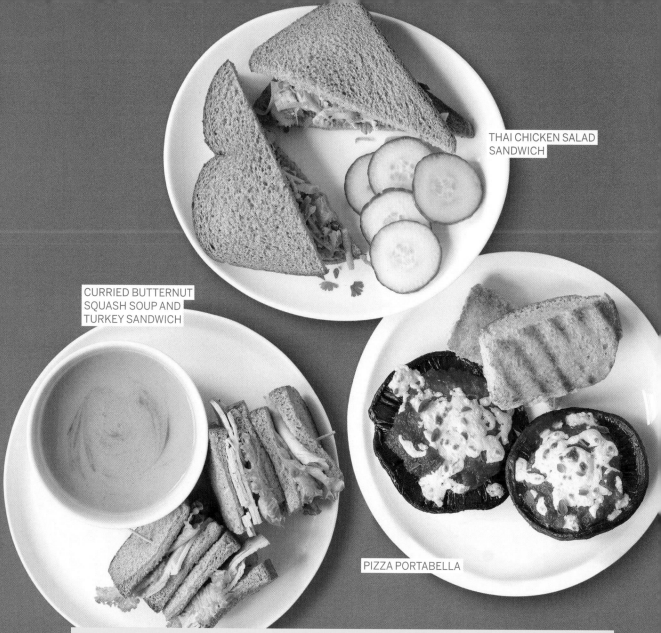

THAI CHICKEN SALAD SANDWICH

CURRIED BUTTERNUT SQUASH SOUP AND TURKEY SANDWICH

PIZZA PORTABELLA

Tasty Snacks
(About 150 calories each; eat two a day.)

- 3 cinnamon graham cracker squares with 2 teaspoons almond butter
- 100-calorie mini bagel with 2 tablespoons hummus and a slice of tomato

- 5-Spice Dip with Pea Pods and Pita. To make dip, mix ¼ cup Greek yogurt and ¼ teaspoon Chinese five-spice blend. Serve with ½ cup pea pods and ½ whole-grain pita, sliced into triangles.
- 100-calorie bag of popcorn mixed with 1 tablespoon peanuts

- 1 cup skim milk blended with ½ banana, 3 teaspoons unsweetened cocoa powder and ice
- 1 small banana topped with 1 teaspoon each peanut butter and melted chocolate and chilled
- 10 baked tortilla chips with ¼ cup black bean dip

Power Lunches (about 400 calories each)

Pizza Portabella
Turn 2 portobello mushroom caps (stems removed) upside down, spread with 6 tablespoons spaghetti sauce and top with 1 ounce shredded part-skim mozzarella cheese. Place on a baking sheet and broil for 10 minutes. Sprinkle with 1 teaspoon dried oregano. Cut a whole-grain roll in half and toast; drizzle with olive oil.

Curried Butternut Squash Soup and Turkey Sandwich
Heat 1 ½ cups prepared butternut squash soup and add ¼ teaspoon curry powder. Spread 2 teaspoons Dijon mustard on 2 slices whole-grain bread; top with 2 ounces low-sodium deli turkey, lettuce and tomato slices.

Nachos Supreme
In a skillet, cook 4 ounces ground turkey with 1 tablespoon taco seasoning. Put 12 baked tortilla chips on a plate; top with cooked turkey mixture, ½ cup canned black beans, rinsed and drained, and ¼ cup shredded light cheddar cheese. Microwave for approximately 1 minute until cheese melts; top with 2 tablespoons salsa and ½ cup shredded lettuce.

Blue Cheese Veggie Burger
Prepare 1 veggie burger according to directions. Place cooked burger on 1 toasted whole-wheat hamburger bun, and top with 1 slice red onion, 2 slices tomato, 1 tablespoon blue cheese crumbles and 1 tablespoon barbecue sauce.

Serve veggie burger with 10 each baby carrots and cherry tomatoes with 1 tablespoon light ranch dressing for dipping.

Cuban Sandwich
Grill 2 ounces low-fat sliced ham in a pan for 4 minutes, turning once. Spread 2 teaspoons mustard on a whole-grain bun and top with ham, 1 slice Swiss cheese and dill pickle slices. Serve with a small apple.

Chunky Greek Salad with Chickpeas
Mix together ½ cup each cucumber, chopped tomato and red and green pepper. Add ½ cup chickpeas, rinsed and drained; 5 Kalamata olives, pitted and sliced; and ¼ red onion, sliced. Toss with 2 tablespoons red wine vinegar and ½ tablespoon olive oil. Sprinkle with 2 tablespoons crumbled reduced-fat feta.

Thai Chicken Salad Sandwich
Whisk together 1 tablespoon peanut butter, 2 tablespoons seasoned rice vinegar and ⅛ teaspoon crushed red pepper until smooth. Stir in ½ cup shredded carrot, 1 tablespoon chopped cilantro and 2 ounces diced, cooked chicken breast. Spread on 2 slices whole-grain bread. Serve with cucumbers.

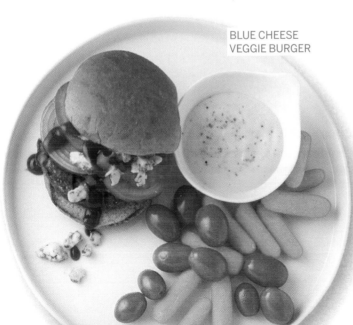
BLUE CHEESE VEGGIE BURGER

Delicious Dinners (about 500 calories each)

Steak Salad with Croutons

Mist a baking sheet and 1 medium potato, cut into cubes, with nonstick cooking spray; sprinkle with salt and pepper to taste. Broil for 20 minutes, turning once. Grill 3½ ounces sirloin steak until it reaches 160°; cut into strips. Top 3 cups chopped romaine lettuce with potatoes, steak, 1 tablespoon blue cheese and 2 tablespoons balsamic vinaigrette.

Drumsticks and Salad

Bake, broil or grill 3 skinless chicken drumsticks until they reach 165°. Mix 3 tablespoons hot sauce and 2 tablespoons trans fat–free margarine and spread it on cooked drumsticks. Toss 1 cup chopped romaine lettuce, ½ cup chopped celery, ½ cup shredded carrot and ½ cup grape tomatoes with 1½ tablespoons light ranch dressing and serve on the side.

Turkey Burger and Fries

Toss 1 sliced medium potato with 1 tablespoon chili powder and salt to taste. Mist a baking sheet and tops of potatoes with nonstick cooking spray. Broil potatoes and 1 lean 4-ounce turkey burger for 20 minutes, turning once. Serve burger on a whole-grain bun with lettuce and tomato slices and fries.

Cheesy Turkey Meatballs

Mix ½ pound lean ground turkey with 1 tablespoon diced onion, 1 teaspoon minced garlic, 1 beaten egg, ¼ cup whole-wheat bread crumbs, 2 tablespoons nonfat milk, 1 teaspoon salt and ½ teaspoon pepper. Form 8 meatballs, placing a ½-inch mozzarella cube in center of each. Mist a baking dish with nonstick cooking spray; bake meatballs 15 minutes at 425°. Sauté 2 minced garlic cloves in 1 teaspoon canola oil 1 minute. Add 2 cups chopped zucchini; cook 5 minutes. Serve 4 meatballs over zucchini and ⅓ cup cooked whole-wheat orzo; top with ½ cup tomato sauce. (Freeze leftovers.)

Chili-Rubbed Shrimp Tacos

Season 10 large raw shrimps with ¼ teaspoon chili powder and a pinch of salt and pepper. Sauté in 1 teaspoon extra-virgin olive oil for 5 to 6 minutes until opaque, turning once. Divide shrimp between 2 whole-wheat tortillas; top with ¼ diced avocado, ¼ cup diced tomato, ¼ cup shredded romaine, 2 tablespoons chopped onion and 1 tablespoon chopped fresh cilantro. Serve with ¼ cup tomatillo salsa.

Smoky Veggie Chili

Combine ½ cup canned pinto beans, rinsed and drained; ½ cup canned black beans, rinsed and drained; ⅔ cup corn; ½ cup fire-roasted diced tomatoes with green chilies; ½ cup tomato sauce; 1 tablespoon barbecue sauce; ¼ teaspoon garlic powder; and ¼ teaspoon chili powder. Bring to a boil. Reduce heat; simmer for 15 minutes. Serve over ½ cup cooked brown rice; top with 2 tablespoons chopped onion and 2 tablespoons shredded low-fat cheddar cheese.

Chicken Satay with Peanut Sauce

Cut a 6-ounce chicken breast into strips; season with salt and pepper. Mist a pan with nonstick cooking spray; saute chicken 6 to 8 minutes, turning once. In a bowl, combine 2 tablespoons peanut butter, 2 tablespoons chicken broth, 2 teaspoons soy sauce, 2 teaspoons lime juice and 2 teaspoons brown sugar. Microwave 5 to 10 seconds and whisk well. In a separate bowl, toss 1 small cucumber, thinly sliced; 2 tablepoons rice wine vinegar; ⅛ teaspoon sugar; and 1 teaspoon chopped mint. Serve alongside chicken and dipping sauce.

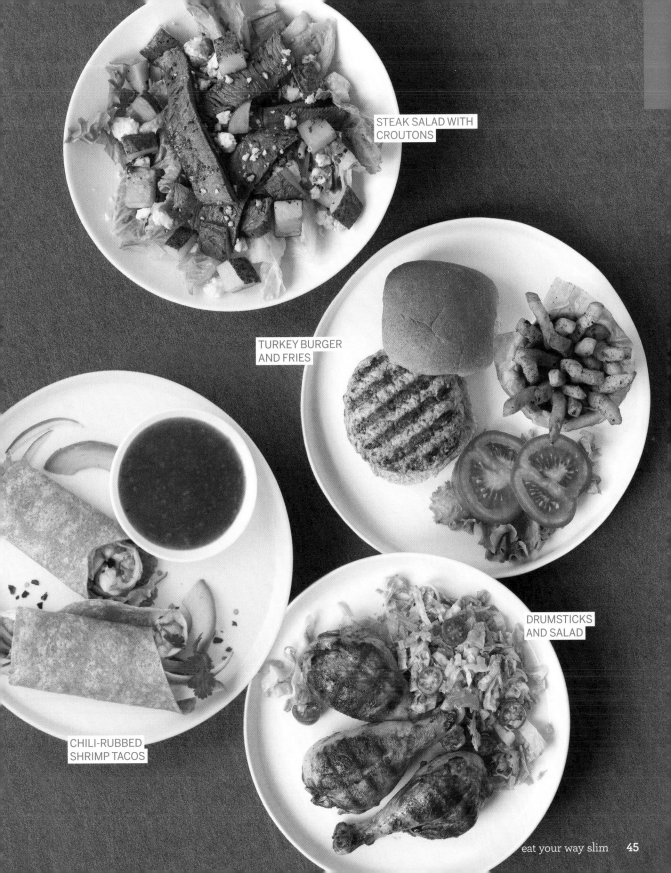

STEAK SALAD WITH CROUTONS

TURKEY BURGER AND FRIES

DRUMSTICKS AND SALAD

CHILI-RUBBED SHRIMP TACOS

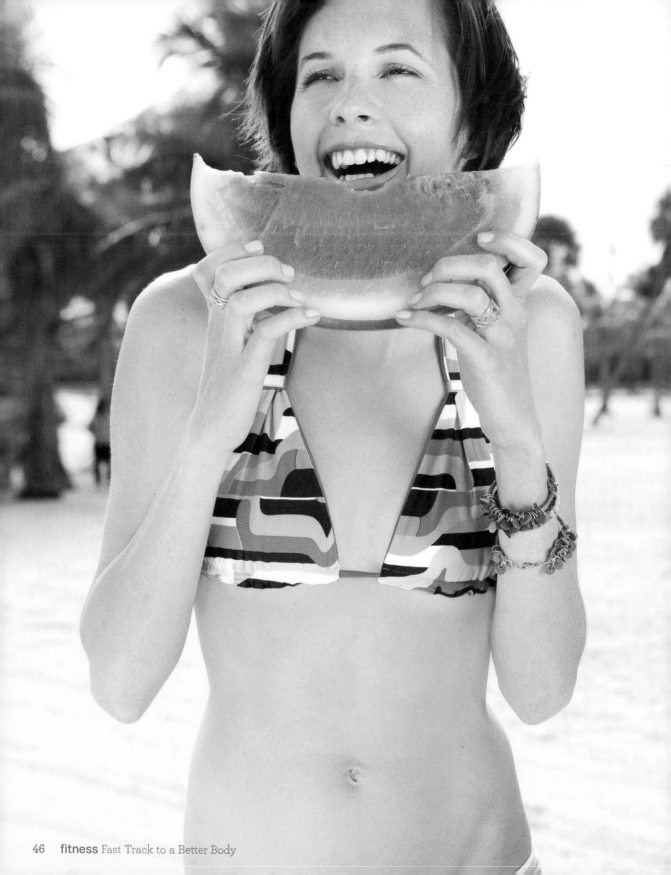

fitness Fast Track to a Better Body

Diet Myths Debunked

Think snacking on celery torches calories? Fresh fruit is better than frozen? See if you've bought into any of these misconceptions—and get the scoop on the truth.

Myth: Dieting shrinks your stomach.

The real deal: The only way to change your stomach's size is with surgery, but you may feel like your stomach has shrunk after you drop pounds. Consistently taking in fewer calories reprograms the hormones and nerve endings that control satiety, so you need less food to feel full. Even though you can't shrink your stomach, you can downsize your appetite.

Myth: Certain foods have "negative" calories.

The real deal: Although there's no such thing as a (calorie) free lunch, there's some truth to this myth. Different foods have different "thermic effects," which is the energy it takes you to digest, absorb, and metabolize them. High-fiber, low-cal foods generally have a higher thermic effect, so celery, with 1.6 grams of fiber and just 16 calories per cup, has become the negative-calorie-food poster child. But the science stops there, because you use only a fraction of those calories to fuel the digestive process (in other words, chomping stalk after stalk is not a workout). If you slim down snacking on celery, it's simply because you're filling your stomach with just a very few calories.

Myth: Sea salt is more nutritious than table salt.

The real deal: Snazzy marketing and trendy varieties, including

Peruvian Pink, Hawaiian and Black, make the Morton's Girl seem a little passé, but the two salts have the same nutritional makeup. Manufacturers of sea salt claim it contains good-for-you trace minerals that are not in table salt, but there's not enough to make a difference to your health. There is one benefit, however: Sea salt has a more intense flavor, so you may be able to get away with using less. Good news, since sodium has long been linked to high blood pressure and heart disease.

Myth: I'll lose weight if I follow a diet based on my blood type.
The real deal: The premise is that some foods contain proteins called lectins that interact with certain blood types and cause weight gain, but there's no scientific evidence to support the claim. Instead, these programs often restrict good-for-you foods that your body needs, such as tomatoes and carrots. Still, don't be surprised if you drop a jeans size on a blood-type diet; whether you're type AB or O, the plan will encourage you to consume whole grains, lean protein and plenty of produce and limit refined carbs and processed snacks. But instead of hopping on the blood type diet bandwagon, why not simply eat healthy without cutting out vitamin- and nutrient-rich foods?

Myth: Sugar makes you fat.
The real deal: It only seems like those Girl Scout cookies go straight to your thighs. Sugar doesn't automatically convert into fat in your body. Repeat after us: Eating too many calories is what makes you gain weight—whether they come from cookies or carrots. But when was the last time you ate too many carrots? Sugary foods tend to be high in calories and easy to overeat, because they make your blood sugar spike. The sudden drop can leave you feeling depleted and hungry.

Myth: Vegetarians are healthier than meat eaters.
The real deal: Sure, eating lots of veggies is healthy. But in gen-

eral, cutting out an entire food group—even if it is one that can be high in saturated fat—is a bad idea. Meat is a key source of iron, which keeps your energy levels up, allows you to think clearly and produces enzymes that fight infection. Moreover, researchers at Pennsylvania State University have shown that iron deficiency increases a woman's risk for postpartum depression. Vegetarians often try to get their iron fix through lentils, beans, fortified cereals and tofu. However, you're still missing some protein. Make sure to eat eggs, dairy products or soy at every meal to get your animal-friendly dose.

Myth: Brown sugar is better than white.
The real deal: The darker-hued variety of the sweet stuff has about five calories less per teaspoon and contains trace amounts of minerals, including calcium, potassium and iron (thanks to the molasses that is added to it). However, such a small amount won't make a difference to your health. Instead of fretting over which kind to sprinkle on your oatmeal, cut back on sugar from beverages and processed foods. According to the USDA, the average American consumes 102 pounds per year, or $\frac{2}{3}$ cup per day. The number-one source? Sweetened drinks (soda, fruit juice and sports drinks).

Myth: Fresh fruit is better than frozen.
The real deal: With shipping and storage, fresh fruit can often sit around for as long as two weeks before it hits your supermarket. During that time, it can lose a lot of its nutrients, especially vitamin C. In contrast, frozen fruit is often picked and frozen at the peak of freshness. It's also a better choice for concocting smoothies. But watch out for frozen fruits in syrup—it packs extra calories.

The Big Fat Truth

You've shied away from eating dietary fat and worked on the treadmill to burn off body fat. But fat, it turns out, can be your friend.

That's right: Women who ate a Mediterranean diet filled with healthy monounsaturated fat lowered their risk of heart disease by 29 percent, according to a study in the journal *Circulation*. Of your total daily calories, 25 to 30 percent should come from fat. The key? Pick good-for-you fats, like those found in the Eat More, Lose More diet, and limit the bad kinds. It's okay if you don't know a saturated from a poly—here's the skinny on which fats to eat and which to avoid.

The Good: Unsaturated Fats

Monounsaturated Fats

What they do: These fats, known as MUFAs, raise good HDL cholesterol, lower bad LDL cholesterol and protect against the buildup of plaque in your arteries. They also help prevent belly fat.

Where you'll find them: In olive oil and olives, canola oil, almonds, cashews, peanuts, peanut butter, sesame seeds and avocados. Check out the Flat Abs Diet in Chapter 6 for an eating plan that incorporates MUFAs from foods like these.

How much you need: Most of the fat you eat should be unsaturated, like MUFAs. Just two to three tablespoons of olive oil a day can raise HDL levels and protect against heart disease.

Polyunsaturated Fats

What they do: In addition to lowering your LDL, these fats contain essential omega-3 fatty acids—which boost brain function and may help strengthen your immune system and improve your mood

—and omega-6 fatty acids, which in small amounts can keep skin and eyes healthy.

Where you'll find them: Omega-3s are primarily in fish like salmon, mackerel and herring, as well as canola oil, flaxseed, walnuts and tofu. Omega-6s are in corn and safflower oil, corn-fed chicken and beef, and farmed fish.

How much you need: Most of the polys you eat should be omega-3s. Too much omega-6 can lead to inflammation, which is linked to heart disease. Trade vegetable oil for olive and canola oils, and eat grass-fed beef and wild-caught fish.

The Bad: Saturated Fats

What they do: They raise cholesterol levels and increase your risk of heart disease.

Where you'll find them: In meat and poultry, in dairy products like cream, butter, and whole and 2 percent milk, and in some plant foods like coconut and palm oil.

How much you need: Limit saturated fat to less than 10 percent of your total daily calories. One easy way to cut back: "Remove any hard fat you can see, such as the skin on chicken," says Christine Gerbstadt, M.D., R.D., a spokesperson for the American Dietetic Association.

The Ugly: Trans Fats

What they do: Made from unsaturated fat that's been chemically altered to prolong the shelf life of packaged foods, trans fats raise bad LDL cholesterol and lower good HDL cholesterol, increasing inflammation throughout the body. "They 100 percent promote heart disease," says Dr. Gerbstadt.

Where you'll find them: In shortening, margarine, doughnuts, french fries, and processed foods such as crackers, cookies, chips and cakes.

How much you need: Zero.

Feed Your Face

Eight diet foods that can make you gorgeous.

Eat for: shiny locks

• Walnuts are packed with omega-3 fatty acids, which keep the scalp flake-free, as well as copper, a mineral that naturally helps strands shine, says nutritionist Lisa Drayer, R.D. Toss a quarter cup into your yogurt.

Eat for: a clear complexion

• One cup of kiwi has more wrinkle-fighting vitamin C than a cup of orange segments—220 percent of your daily value, says Allison Tannis, a beauty expert.

• The hue of a sweet potato comes from beta-carotene (it has about as much as a carrot), which is converted into skin-softening vitamin A in the body, Tannis says. Have one cup of it baked to get a healthy dose.

• Sip a cup of hot cocoa to get twice the amount of antioxidant flavanols as you would from a glass of red wine, Drayer says. They increase blood flow to the skin for added radiance.

• Spinach helps fend off sunburns. The vitamin A in this dark leafy green protects skin from UV damage and ensures healthy cell turnover, which keeps you looking radiant. Steam and toss spinach with garlic, lemon juice and olive oil, or use leaves to fill out a sandwich.

Eat for: stronger, whiter teeth

• That cup of plain low-fat yogurt you have as a snack offers half your daily need of enamel-building calcium and has tooth-strengthening phosphorous, says Drayer.

• Onions prevent cavities: They contain sulfur, a powerful

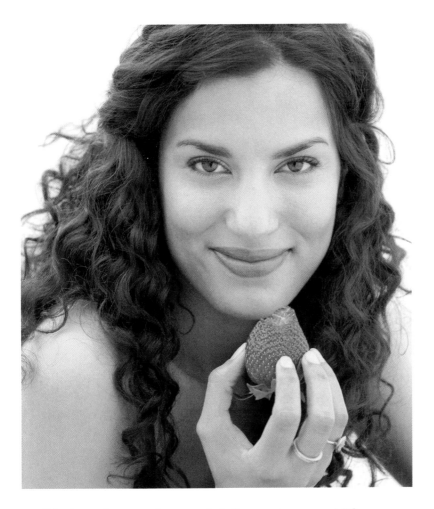

antibiotic, and quercetin, an anti-inflammatory agent. These compounds have been shown to kill various types of bacteria, like *Streptococcus mutans,* which can contribute to tooth decay. Raw onions are more potent than cooked ones, so use them in salads or stir them into guacamole, salsa and other dips.

• Brush, floss . . . and snack on strawberries? Yup. It turns out that the fruit contains salicylic acid, a natural tooth whitener. "Strawberries are a potent plaque fighter, and they actually contain a mild bleaching agent that's used in many commercial products," says Janice Cox, a beauty expert. Puree a handful of fresh strawberries and add it to iced green tea.

Conquer Cravings

Even with the best, most balanced diet, sometimes the urge to splurge is overwhelming. Squelch it with these sneaky strategies.

Hit the road. If you're pining for a peanut butter cup, take a hike. In a recent study in the journal *Appetite,* a 15-minute stroll reduced cravings in chocoholics—perhaps because exercise boosts levels of the feel-good brain chemical serotonin. Another study found that exercise may release satiety hormones that keep your appetite in check for 24 hours!

Get busy. Try distracting yourself from thoughts of cookies and candy for 20 minutes (the usual length of a craving) by chatting on the phone or running an errand.

Eat protein. Ghrelin, a hormone that's produced in the gut, normally spikes before mealtime. The bigger the spike, the hungrier you are. But research shows that eating protein curbs ghrelin, so reach for protein-rich snacks between meals (for example, apple slices with peanut butter or low-fat cheese).

Stay strong. After ovulation (about 14 days after the first day of your period), the hormone progesterone increases, which can lead to decreased energy and heightened cravings for calories, fat and sugar. Consider days 14 to 28 of your cycle "red alert days," when it's most important to have healthy snacks, such as popcorn with a sprinkling of Parmesan or Greek yogurt with a smidge of honey and fresh berries, at the ready and not skip your workout.

Give in (sort of). Trade your usual picks for the lower-calorie, nutrient-packed options on the opposite page.

Your Don't-Cheat Sheet

INSTEAD OF...	HAVE...	WHAT YOU GET...
• 3-ounce regular hamburger (248 calories, 21 g fat, 8 g saturated fat)	• 3-ounce salmon burger (120 calories, 5 g fat, 1 g saturated fat)	• Lose: 128 calories, 16 g fat, 7 g saturated fat • Gain: A healthy serving of omega-3 fatty acids
• One 2-ounce candy bar, like Snickers (271 calories, 14 g fat, 5 g saturated fat)	• 1 ounce peanuts (166 calories, 14 g fat, 2 g saturated fat)	• Lose: 105 calories, 3 g saturated fat • Gain: More than 25 mcg of folate
• 1-ounce bag Lay's Classic potato chips (150 calories, 10 g fat, 1 g saturated fat)	• ½ cup raw carrots with ¼ cup hummus (129 calories, 6 g fat, 1 g saturated fat)	• Lose: 21 calories, 4 g fat • Gain: Total daily requirement for Vitamin A
• 1 medium baked potato with 2 tablespoons sour cream (221 calories, 6 g fat, 5 g saturated fat)	• 1 sweet potato with 1½ cups bell peppers and broccoli, sautéed in ½ tablespoons olive oil (207 cals, 7 g fat, 1 g saturated fat)	• Lose: 14 calories, 4 g saturated fat • Gain: More than double the RDA for vitamin C and vitamin A, plus phytonutrients and folate
• 1 large plain bagel with 2 tablespoons cream cheese (461 calories, 12 g fat, 5 g saturated fat)	• 2 slices whole-grain toast with 1½ tablespoons peanut butter (293 calories, 14 g fat, 3 g saturated fat)	• Lose: 168 calories, 2 g saturated fat • Gain: Phytonutrients, folate and satisfying protein
• 2 pieces French toast with 3 tablespoons syrup (455 calories, 14 g fat, 4 g saturated fat)	• 2-egg omelet made with vegetable-oil cooking spray and ¼ cup chopped tomatoes (or other veggie); whole-grain toast (227 calories, 11 g fat, 3 g saturated fat)	• Lose: 228 calories, 3 g fat • Gain: 19 mcg selenium, 11 mcg folate, 5 mg vitamin C, a little vitamin D, phytonutrients • Bonus: Use omega-3 enriched eggs

Stay Motivated!

Practice these tried-and-true mind tricks to make sure you don't lose your thinspiration.

Save up your willpower. A recent study published in *Psychology & Health* suggests that people have a finite amount of self-control, and that it can run dry. To keep from depleting your inner strength during the first week you start a diet, avoid tempting situations. Plan to have dinner at home instead of at restaurants; don't walk by the doughnut shop on your way to work. And squeeze in a workout first thing in the morning, before your motivation runs out.

Plan for slipups. Let's face it, sometimes you're going to eat ice cream or skip cardio class. Slipups are inevitable; it's how you respond that matters. Don't beat yourself up; instead go through your takeout menus and highlight five healthy options for next time. Set up an alternative workout for no-gym days, even if it's simply running around the block or doing lunges in your living room.

Stick with the scale. Love it and you'll probably lose pounds. In a study at the University of Minnesota, Twin Cities, of 3,026 adults who were watching their waistlines, those who weighed themselves frequently lost more weight over two years or regained fewer pounds. This research backs up the benefits of daily weigh-ins, but weekly may do the trick: Three-quarters of the successful long-term slimmers listed in the National Weight Control Registry step on the scale at least once a week. "Plateaus are part of the process," says Kim H. Miller, Ph.D., associate professor of health promotion at the University of Kentucky in Lexington. Boost your morale in the meantime by giving yourself credit for how much better your clothes fit and for improving your overall health.

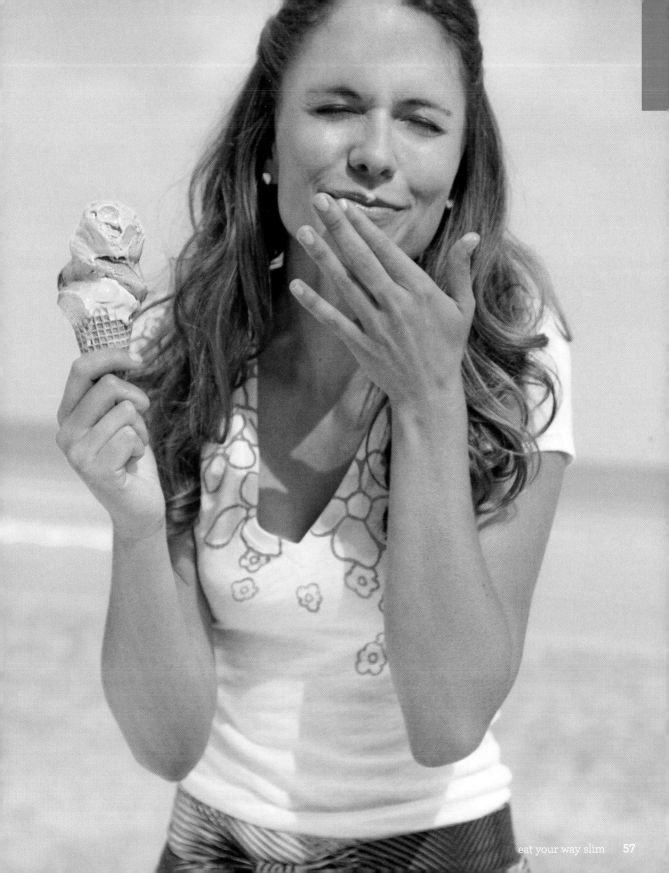

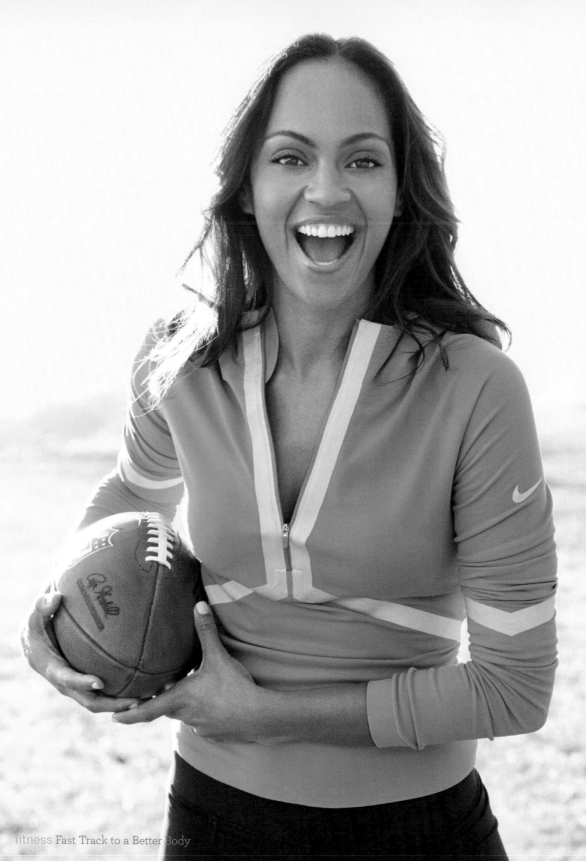

CHAPTER 3

sweat off stress

SHED POUNDS, GAIN ENERGY AND
STRENGTHEN YOUR IMMUNE SYSTEM
SIMPLY BY LEARNING HOW TO CHILL.

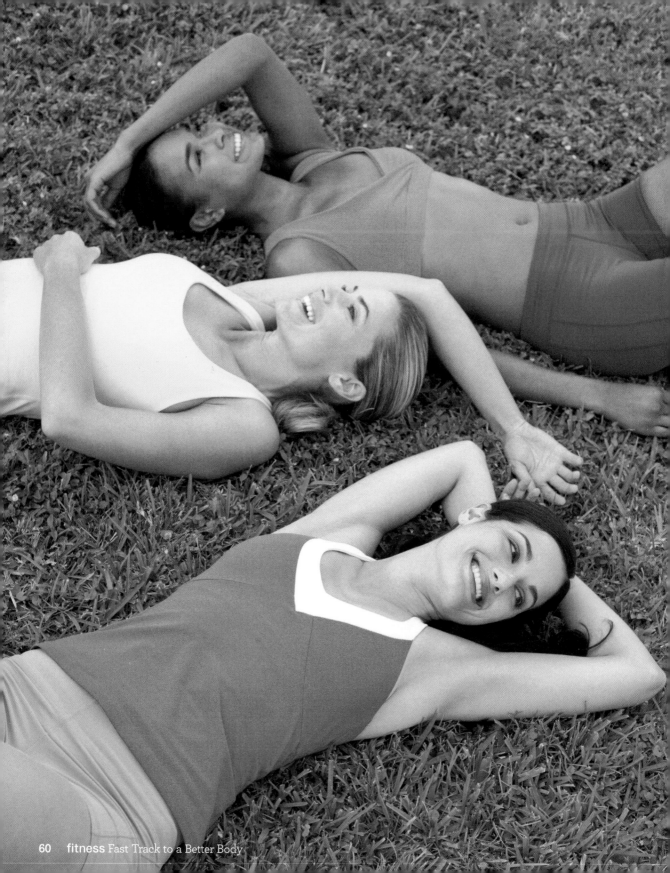

F eeling overwhelmed? You're not alone. According to a new study from the American Psychological Association, 75 percent of us are stressed out. Unfortunately, stress doesn't just mess with your head. It actually messes with your waistline. When your body faces intense pressure, it increases the production of cortisol, a hormone that increases the flow of glucose into the bloodstream in order to boost your energy levels. You crave high-fat, high-sugar foods in response, and cortisol encourages those extra calories to be stored in your abs. The result: belly fat. If your stress is ongoing (money troubles or long hours at the office every day), the cortisol keeps cranking out and your waist begins to expand.

It seems unfair that the consequence of being stressed out is belly fat, which makes you more stressed, but it gets worse. Ab fat (aka dangerous visceral fat) wraps itself around your internal organs, where it can do serious damage. (Non-stress-related fat tends to lie just below the skin surface, where, though unattractive, it poses less of a health risk; you'll read more about both types of ab fat in Chapter 6.) "Stress is associated with every chronic disease we know, including heart disease, diabetes, depression and some cancers," says Jill Goldstein, Ph.D., director of research at the Connors Center for Women's Health and Gender Biology at Brigham and Women's Hospital in Boston.

....

Did You Know? LEVELS OF THE STRESS HORMONE CORTISOL DIP AS MUCH AS 25 PERCENT AFTER JUST ONE 50-MINUTE YOGA SESSION, ACCORDING TO THE CENTER OF INTEGRATIVE MEDICINE AT THOMAS JEFFERSON UNIVERSITY IN PHILADELPHIA.

Although you experience it as an emotion, stress response is largely a physical one. "You get into an argument with your boyfriend, or you're harboring anxiety about work, and your brain responds by cranking out powerful hormones that increase your blood pressure and heart rate," explains Monika Fleshner, Ph.D., a professor at the Center for Neuroscience Department of Integrative Physiology at University of Colorado, Boulder. Often, you can't control anxiety-inducing situations. "There will always be stressors," says Fleshner. "They become damaging to your health if they're repeated—and you can't manage your response."

Conventional wisdom suggests you're just a downward-dog, deep-breath, good-night's-sleep away from having a stress-free life. And these things do help. But according to the latest research, an equally effective antidote to stress is to rev your body up with exercise. Scientists now believe that regular physical activity—particularly cardio—actually "remodels" the brain to make it more resistant to stress hormones. Princeton University researchers recently compared the brain cells of exercisers following a long-term fitness program with non-exercisers. Turns out, the "brains on exercise" morphed over time into a biochemically calm state that remained steady under stress. Even moderate amounts of physical activity, such as brisk walking several times a week, appear to have a protective effect, according to a University of Houston study.

The Fitness Fix

So how does exercise lower your stress levels? Cardio sessions, such as walking, biking or jogging, help the heart pump more blood to the brain. Increased blood flow means more oxygen; more oxygen means better-nourished brain cells. Plus, scientists have discovered that a vigorous workout boosts the production of a protein that fortifies brain cells from breaking down when exposed to stress.

The catch: You have to keep up with regular exercise sessions to maintain the levels of the stress-proofing protein in your body. And the longer you stick with it, the more stress protection you'll get: In one study, people who ran regularly for three weeks all showed a drop in stress and anxiety levels, but those who ran for six weeks had a significantly greater reduction in stress hormones. In other words, the more consistent you are with your workouts, the more you are rewarded with stress-fighting power.

Of course, exercise doesn't need to be high-impact cardio in order for it to help de-stress your life. Other research shows that yoga and routines that involve gentle stretching of your muscles and ligaments can be beneficial in producing chemicals that protect your brain from stress. Moreover, these workouts instill a sense of calmness that can help you lower your blood pressure and heart rate, both of which rise when you're feeling stressed and set you up for serious heart problems down the road.

Ready to reap the benefits of a stress-free life? Just turn the page to get started now.

Calm On

Get instant aah with these soothe moves.

Breathe right. "Most of us take short, shallow breaths when we're stressed," says Ann Pardo, director of life management at Canyon Ranch Spa in Tucson, Arizona. This decreases your blood oxygen levels. Instead, inhale deeply through your nose for a count of five; exhale through your mouth for the same.

Strike a pose. Lie on your back with legs propped in an L position against a wall, hands on the floor above your head. This pose reverses the normal downward flow of blood and stretches the neck, back and leg muscles, to help relax you.

Sniff a mango. You've probably heard that the scent of lavender has a soothing effect. Now scientists in Japan have found that compounds in mango produce the same stress-reducing benefits. (When you're done inhaling, go ahead and eat it—mangoes are full of good-for-you vitamins C and E.)

Choose decaf. Without sugar. Both caffeine and the sweet stuff cause an almost-instant spike in energy levels, followed by a steep decline when they wear off. Keep your energy levels constant by limiting caffeine intake to one caffeinated beverage a day (that includes tea, coffee and soda).

Hit the mat. Yoga's emphasis on breathing, mediation and relaxation has been linked in studies with heart-healthy benefits, such as reduced stress. "Slow and steady methods, such as Iyengar, do the trick; because ashtanga and power yoga are faster, they lack enough mindfulness to give the relaxation effect," says Cyndi Lee, a FITNESS advisory board member and owner of Om Yoga in New

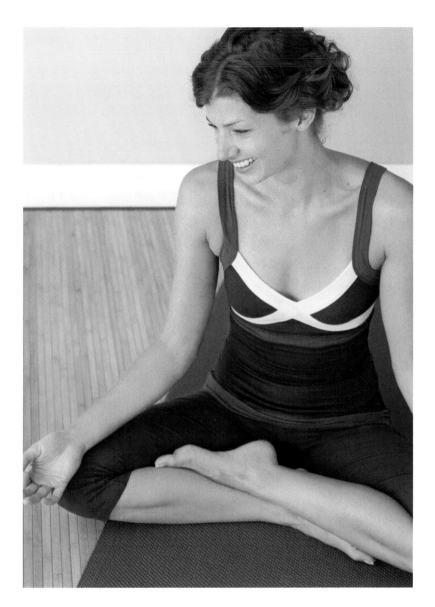

York City. "For best results, breathe deeply but quietly as you go, and only through your nose."

Feel the heat. Take a shower before bed and turn up the water temperature for the last minute. Stepping from the steamy stall into the cool room air causes your body to release melatonin, a sleep-inducing hormone.

Ease your arms. We carry a lot of tension in our forearms (you can thank your frantic texting habit when you're feeling anxious). To relax, place your forearm on a flat desk, palm down. Gently knead tense areas using your opposite elbow. Switch sides and repeat.

Make peace with your boss. A Swedish study found that women in anxiety-inducing relationships—at work or at home—had more stress and sleep difficulties than those in positive relationships.

Tense and release. While sitting at your desk (or lying in bed at home) try to contract and release each area of your body, starting with your shoulders and working down to your toes. The goal is to focus on one spot at a time—while you're tensing your shoulders, for instance, the rest of you should be relaxed.

Take a break. Even if you don't have the time or the money for a full-fledged vacation, block out 20 minutes on your daily calendar that are just for you. No texting, no TV, no kids. Find a quiet place to sit and, well, enjoy the silence. Close your eyes and focus on the sound of your breath. You will return to the real world refreshed.

Play cards. Hello computer solitaire! Research shows that distracting yourself with games that activate your brain's recall and processing areas makes it virtually impossible for you to simultaneously ruminate over whatever is stressing you out.

Play some music. Studies show that soothing music goes a long way to easing anxiety. Make a playlist of happy-go-lucky songs to plug into next time life starts bringing you down.

Treat yourself. Eating about an ounce and a half of dark chocolate every day for two weeks reduced levels of stress hormones in people feeling highly anxious.

Roll out the kinks. Tight back muscles are a classic side effect of stress. To get relief, place a tennis ball between a wall and your upper back, and push sore areas against it. Bend your knees a few degrees, then straighten them, allowing the ball to roll up and down your back while giving gentle pressure to areas that need relaxing. (Stick to the muscles; steer clear of your spine.) For your lower back, lie on the floor, knees bent. Place your fists, knuckles up, under tense areas, and rock back and forth.

Hit the pool. New research shows that swimming can help lower cortisol levels for both chronic and acute stress situations.

Catch some rays. Fifteen minutes of direct sunlight a day is enough to give your vitamin D levels a boost. Wear sunscreen if you're outside any longer than that. Vitamin D works as a natural antidote to depression and anxiety.

Call a friend. Good moods are contagious. Talk to a friend who always sees the glass half full, and ask her about her day. Hearing her enthusiasm and positive energy will rub off on you, and you'll get a new perspective.

Take note. Every time you feel yourself getting tense, jot down the time of day, likely cause and how you feel. Journaling is an effective tool because it forces you to get specific about what's stressing you out, so you can come up with a plan of action to deal with it.

Eat melon. An antioxidant found in melon has been shown to reduce people's perceived stress and fatigue levels, according to a report in *Nutrition Journal*.

Sip some tea. Green tea is packed with powerful antioxidants that help protect your body from the damaging effects of stress.

Laugh a little. Watch a funny movie, read a humorous book or just force a chuckle for no good reason. The very act of laughing encourages your body to increase the production of feel-good chemicals that help you fight off stress, research shows.

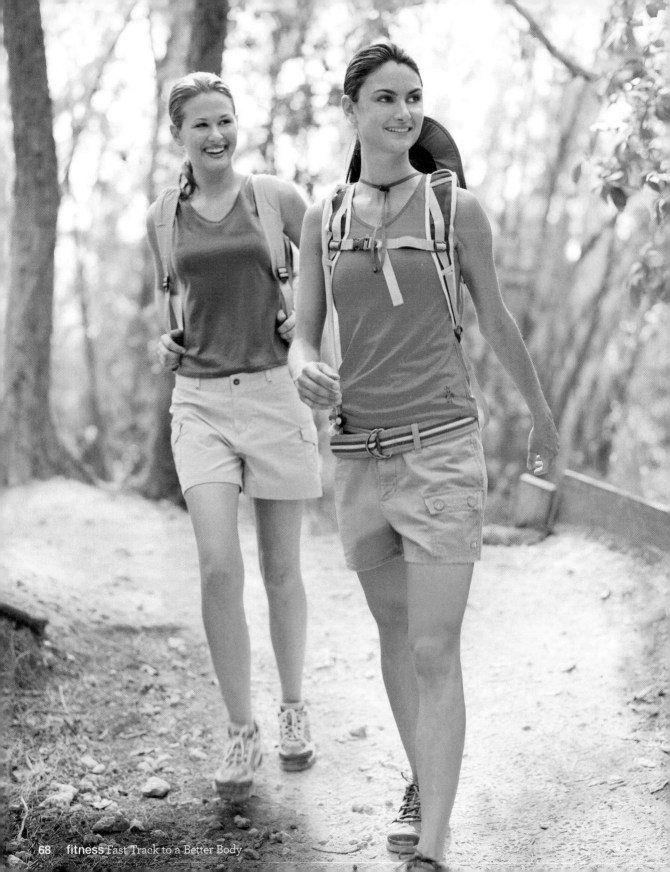

Walk Away Your Worries

Walking is great exercise; done right, it's also a great stress reliever. Incorporate these techniques into your next outing and feel the difference in your energy.

Find your move groove. Anytime you're walking, tune into the pattern of your arms swinging in rhythm with your feet, says psychologist Nina Smiley, Ph.D., coauthor of *The Three Minute Meditator*. "It puts you in a meditative state that can be as restful as a good nap," Smiley says.

Count your steps. Repeat "one, two, one, two" as you stride, picturing the numbers each time, says James Rippe, M.D., a cardiologist in Shrewsbury, Massachusetts. Walkers who used this tactic instantly reduced their stress levels, his research found. One possible reason: Counting forces you to focus on the present, leaving less room for your brain to worry about the future.

See green. A walk in nature lowers stress levels significantly more than pounding the pavement around town, reports a recent study in the journal *Environment and Behavior*. Take your stroll to the park or hit the trails anytime you need an extra dose of relief.

Stretch your breath. Take longer, slower exhales than inhales as you stride, suggests David Coppel, Ph.D., a sports psychologist in Kirkland, Washington. By focusing on specific breathing patterns, you will shift your mind from anxiety-producing "what if" thoughts about the future and think only about the here and now.

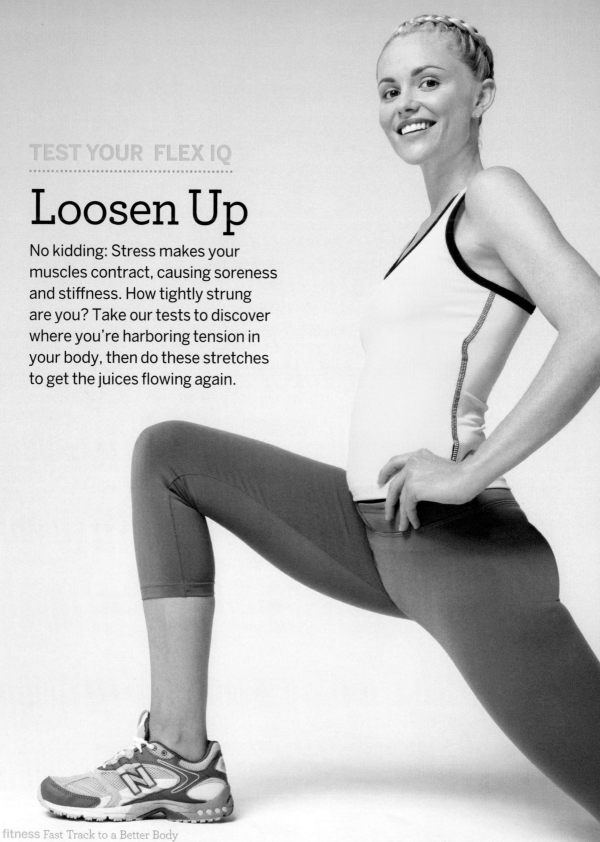

Loosen Up

No kidding: Stress makes your muscles contract, causing soreness and stiffness. How tightly strung are you? Take our tests to discover where you're harboring tension in your body, then do these stretches to get the juices flowing again.

SHOULDERS AND CHEST

Sitting stooped over a desk as well as rarely having to reach overhead means that chest muscles are continually restricted. Loosening up the chest and shoulders will help you reach behind easier to do things like clasp your bra.

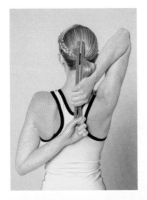

The Test

With left hand, hold a ruler so left thumb is just at the one-inch mark. Bend left arm behind back so ruler points toward head. Now reach right hand up and over right shoulder, grabbing ruler as close to left hand as you can. To measure, pull ruler up with right hand without moving fingers. Write down the number your hand has reached and subtract an inch to get the results for the left shoulder. (You can also try this test without a ruler to see if you can touch or clasp hands.) Switch sides and repeat to test your right shoulder.

- **GOOD** (3 points): Hands touch or are within 3 to 5 inches of each other.
- **FAIR** (2 points): Hands are within 6 to 8 inches of each other.
- **POOR** (1 point): Hands are more than 8 inches apart.

SCORE: Left Side_____ Right Side_____

Stretch It Out

GOALPOST Stand in a doorway and bring left arm directly out to side. Place left forearm against wall to left of doorway, elbow bent 90 degrees at shoulder level. Press left palm and forearm against wall for 5 counts; release. Do 5 reps. Switch sides; repeat.

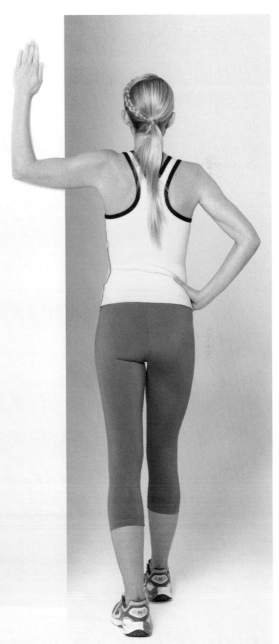

OBLIQUES

Tight obliques and less range of motion in your lower back tend to go hand in hand, so just stretching your back might not be enough, experts say.

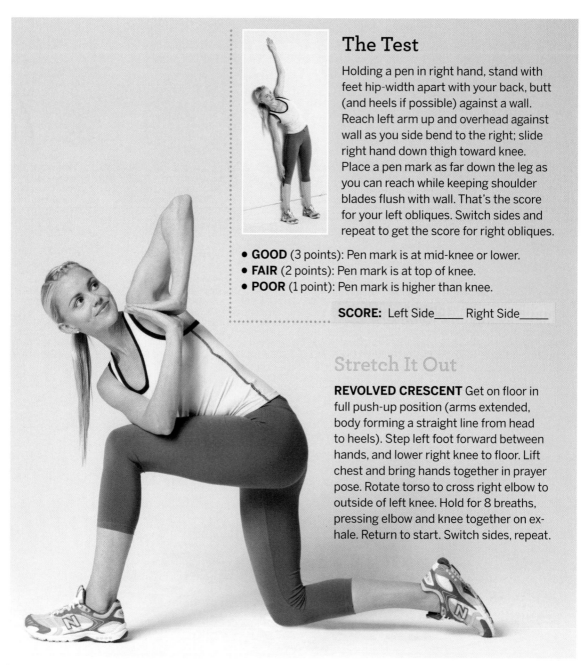

The Test

Holding a pen in right hand, stand with feet hip-width apart with your back, butt (and heels if possible) against a wall. Reach left arm up and overhead against wall as you side bend to the right; slide right hand down thigh toward knee. Place a pen mark as far down the leg as you can reach while keeping shoulder blades flush with wall. That's the score for your left obliques. Switch sides and repeat to get the score for right obliques.

- **GOOD** (3 points): Pen mark is at mid-knee or lower.
- **FAIR** (2 points): Pen mark is at top of knee.
- **POOR** (1 point): Pen mark is higher than knee.

SCORE: Left Side_____ Right Side_____

Stretch It Out

REVOLVED CRESCENT Get on floor in full push-up position (arms extended, body forming a straight line from head to heels). Step left foot forward between hands, and lower right knee to floor. Lift chest and bring hands together in prayer pose. Rotate torso to cross right elbow to outside of left knee. Hold for 8 breaths, pressing elbow and knee together on exhale. Return to start. Switch sides, repeat.

LOWER BACK

Our spines are built to move, so static, everyday activities like driving and standing on line eventually pull on the discs in your lower back, and that's what hurts. Proper stretches keep you mobile and help prevent this ouch.

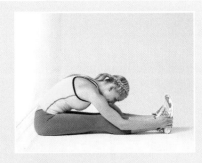

The Test

Sit on floor with back and head against wall, legs extended, knees pressing against floor, feet flexed. Rounding the spine, extend arms forward toward toes by hinging from hips.

- **GOOD** (3 points): Hands can reach ankles or feet.
- **FAIR** (2 points): Hands can reach mid-shin or just above ankle.
- **POOR** (1 point): Hands can only reach area between knee and mid-shin.

SCORE: _____

Stretch It Out

DOWNWARD DOG Start on floor on all fours, then tuck toes under and press hips back and up toward ceiling as you step feet back a few times to form an inverted V, balancing on palms and feet. Exhale, let head drop and release neck to lengthen spine. Hold for 8 to 10 breaths. Lower to knees and sit back on heels. Do 3 to 5 reps.

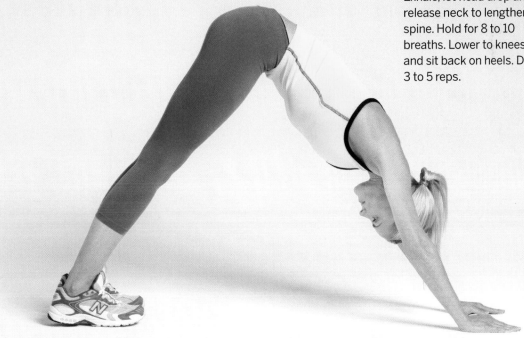

HIPS

When your thighs and hip flexors, the muscles that help lift up the legs, are tight, they may prevent you from lowering fully as you squat down.

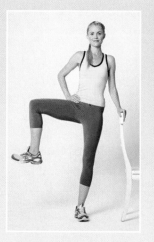

The Test

Stand with feet hip-width apart, left hand holding the back a chair for balance. Bend right knee up to hip height, then bring it directly out to right side. Switch legs and repeat to determine score for left hip.

- **GOOD** (3 points): Thigh is parallel to floor; knee is directly out to the side.
- **FAIR** (2 points): Thigh is parallel; knee is slightly in front of body.
- **POOR** (1 point): Thigh is lower than parallel; knee is slightly in front of body.

SCORE: Left Side_____ Right Side_____

Stretch It Out

LOW LUNGE From downward dog (see previous page), step right foot forward between hands. Lower left knee to floor and press hips forward while lifting torso up as you extend arms overhead. Hold for 8 to 10 breaths. Place palms back on floor on either side of right foot and step back into downward dog. Switch legs, repeat. Do 3 to 5 reps per leg.

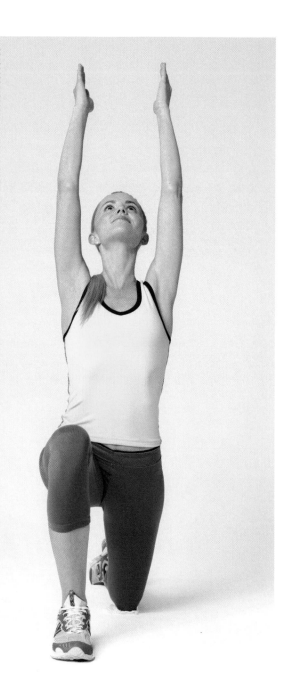

HAMSTRINGS

Calling all office workers: Make it a point to get up and walk around at least once every half hour. Otherwise, hamstrings remain shortened and get stiff.

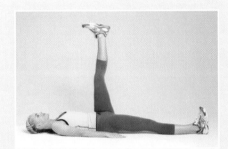

The Test

Lie faceup and lift left leg 90 degrees. Try to straighten left knee, without moving thigh. Switch legs and repeat.

- **GOOD** (3 points): Leg is straight.
- **FAIR** (2 points): Knee is bent 20 degrees.
- **POOR** (1 point): Knee is bent more than 20 degrees.

SCORE: Left Side_____ Right Side_____

Stretch It Out

JACKKNIFE Sit on floor with legs extended in front of you. With back flat, extend arms toward your toes to the point of tension and hold for 15 to 30 seconds. Straighten back up and extend arms toward toes again, this time rounding your back; hold for 15 to 30 seconds. Alternate between a flat and rounded back 4 more times.

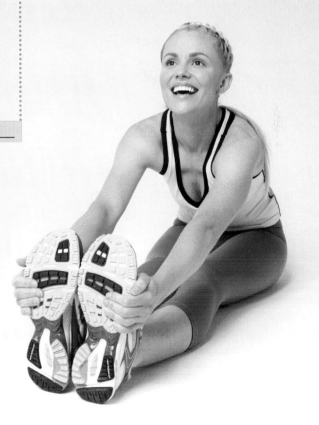

INNER THIGHS

If you sit with your legs crossed all the time, you make your inner thigh muscles steely. Too much of that can cause tension and pain in your knees.

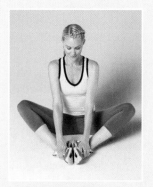

The Test

Sit on floor with knees bent, legs together and feet flat. Lower knees out to sides as far as possible while keeping soles together. Clasp feet with both hands and pull heels as close to body as possible.

- **GOOD** (3 points): Heels are 4 inches from groin.
- **FAIR** (2 points): Heels are 5 to 8 inches from groin.
- **POOR** (1 point): Heels are 9 or more inches from groin.

SCORE: _____

Stretch It Out

MODIFIED FROG Kneel on floor, sitting butt on heels, and fold upper body over thighs, arms stretched forward. Separate knees as widely as you comfortably can. On an exhale, crawl upper body forward without lifting torso (as if you were going to lie on belly), until elbows are bent 90 degrees directly below shoulders. Hold for 8 to 10 breaths. Return to start. Repeat 4 times.

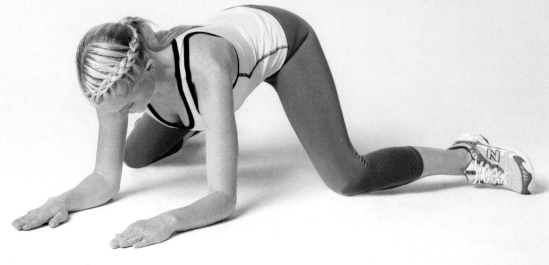

CALVES

Wearing high heels puts your feet in a downward-slanting position that automatically shortens calf muscles. Too much tip-toe strolling over time causes those muscles to remain short even when you're in flats.

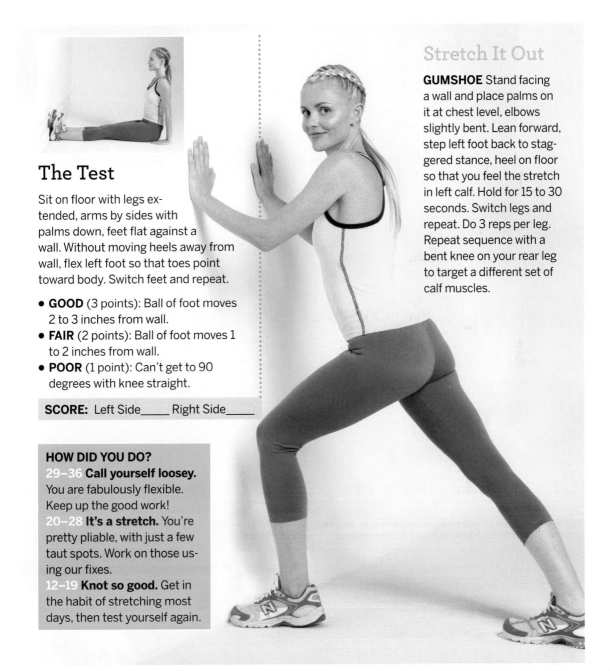

The Test

Sit on floor with legs extended, arms by sides with palms down, feet flat against a wall. Without moving heels away from wall, flex left foot so that toes point toward body. Switch feet and repeat.

- **GOOD** (3 points): Ball of foot moves 2 to 3 inches from wall.
- **FAIR** (2 points): Ball of foot moves 1 to 2 inches from wall.
- **POOR** (1 point): Can't get to 90 degrees with knee straight.

SCORE: Left Side_____ Right Side_____

HOW DID YOU DO?
29–36 Call yourself loosey. You are fabulously flexible. Keep up the good work!
20–28 It's a stretch. You're pretty pliable, with just a few taut spots. Work on those using our fixes.
12–19 Knot so good. Get in the habit of stretching most days, then test yourself again.

Stretch It Out

GUMSHOE Stand facing a wall and place palms on it at chest level, elbows slightly bent. Lean forward, step left foot back to staggered stance, heel on floor so that you feel the stretch in left calf. Hold for 15 to 30 seconds. Switch legs and repeat. Do 3 reps per leg. Repeat sequence with a bent knee on your rear leg to target a different set of calf muscles.

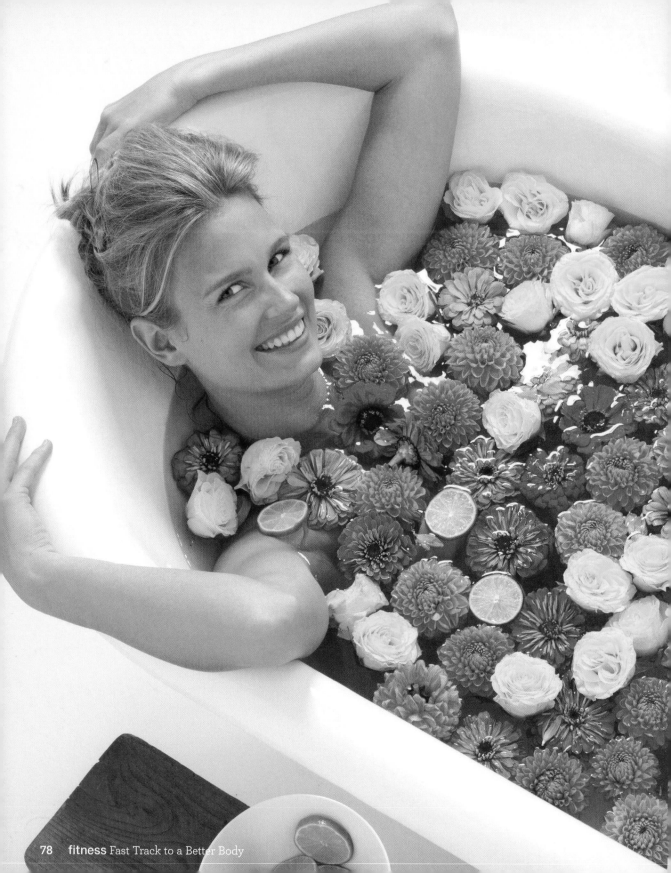

Spa Tricks That De-Stress

Tension can take a real toll on your hair and skin. These seven simple at-home secrets will give your mood—and looks—an instant lift.

Float away frazzle. Taking a bath before bed can help you snooze better, notes a study in the journal *Sleep*. Add a few drops of bath oil or a moisturizing fizzy ball. For a more organic feel, toss in flower heads, such as those from roses and dahlias, and lime slices (as many as you like) while the tub is filling. The oils of the buds moisturize skin, and the vitamin C–rich fruit acts as an astringent, says Gerard Bodeker, author of *Health and Beauty from the Rainforest*.

Find "mist" opportunities. Go from dry to dewy in a spritz. "Floral and herbal waters hydrate skin and keep it glowing," says Terri Lawton, a Los Angeles–based holistic skin-care and wellness expert. Try a premade version like Jurlique Rosewater Balancing Mist, or make your own: Add 1/6 cup dried lavender and 1/2 teaspoon dried sage to 1 cup boiling water, says Marina Valmy, director of New York City's Christine Valmy Skincare. Remove from heat, add 25 rose petals (one large flower) and steep for two hours. Drain the mixture through a coffee filter, then refrigerate in a spray bottle.

Rub off wrinkles. A face massage not only feels wonderful, "it also relaxes muscle tension—smoothing lines—and increases luminosity," says Shelley Bawiec, global skin-care education director for cosmetics company Aveda. Apply a thin layer of lotion to your face, place your palms against your cheeks and rub in fast up-and-down motions, Bawiec instructs. Repeat along your forehead. Next,

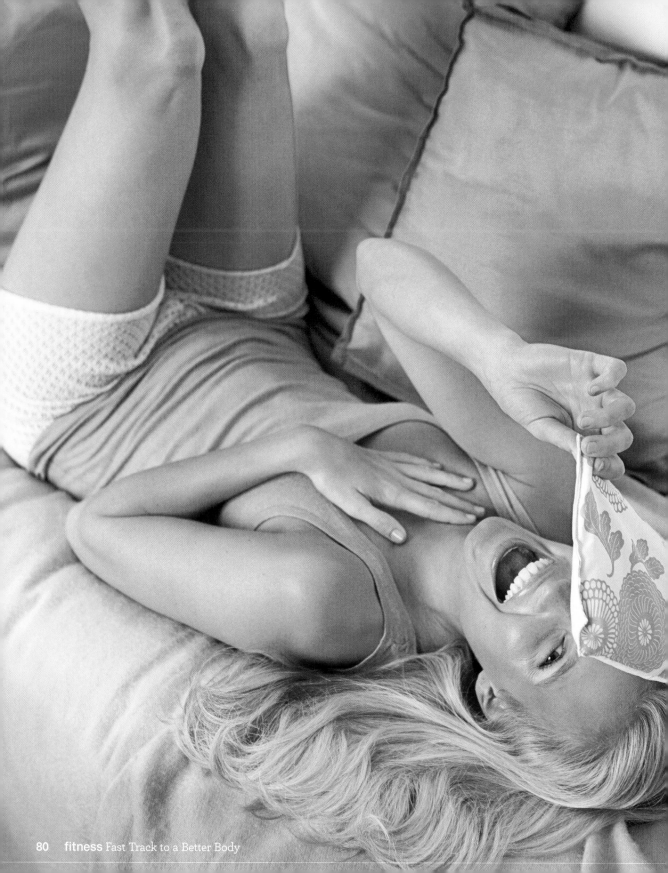

use your index and middle fingers to make small circular motions against the sides of your nose and around your mouth. Finally, press down on the area just under your brows and above the bridge of your nose for three seconds.

Sip super water. Get your eight glasses a day the spa way by adding 5 mint leaves and 10 thin cucumber slices to a pitcher of water, suggests Pam Ouellet, spa director of the Willow Stream Spa at the Fairmont Banff Springs in Alberta, Canada. Mint oil helps flush away complexion-dulling toxins, and vitamins A and C in cucumbers keep skin healthy.

Paint one on. Use an artist's fan brush (available at art supply stores), not your fingers, to apply a face mask. The bristles lightly exfoliate, helping the mask's ingredients penetrate deeper. Mash half a banana and combine it with one tablespoon each orange juice and honey, says Sharon Ronen, owner of Skin Haven Spa Studio & WellSpa in Los Angeles. Apply and rinse after 15 minutes.

Treat your feet. Fill a basin halfway with warm water, then add a few river rocks ($14.99 for 10, rubrocks.com). "Press your soles down on them, or use one to knead away pain caused by running," Hittleman says. After, paint your toenails a deep blue, green or lavender. "These spa colors project feelings of calm," adds Craig Fossella, founder of Tru Spa in San Francisco.

Chill out. Spas and gyms offer cool, eucalyptus-scented cloths in their locker rooms. "The scent helps relax your breathing and clear your mind," says Carol Espel, national director of group fitness and Pilates for Equinox Fitness clubs. Keep a supply on hand: Add 12 drops of eucalyptus oil (available at health food stores) to a sink full of cool water, Espel says. Dip each washcloth into the H_2O, wring out, fold in half, roll up and store in the fridge. After an intense workout, unroll a cloth and lay it over your face until you feel calm.

What to Eat to Beat Tension

Put an end to those mindless munchies in one step.

When you're under the gun and looking for an outlet for your anxiety, if you're like many women, you probably turn to food. Cold comfort, as it turns out: Chowing down won't give you the fix you're searching for, but it will cause you to pack on pounds. Stress actually dampens the brain's response to food and satiety, making it easier to overeat, says a recent study.

Not only that, but "when you're stressed, you're thinking about a million things at once, so your hand is going from the bag of chips to your mouth without your brain really registering that you're eating," explains Evelyn Tribole, R.D., coauthor of *Intuitive Eating*. To break the cycle, Tribole says, measure out a portion of the food you're craving, "put it on a plate, and sit at the table. Take a few deep breaths; focus on the treat in front of you and savor every bite." Which foods to choose for fastest stress relief? Try these:

Shrimp: Omega-3 fatty acids in shellfish may boost your mood by reducing stress hormones, like cortisol. People who ate three to four ounces a day lowered their risk of anxiety, depression and stress by 30 percent, according to research from the University of Las Palmas de Gran Canaria in Spain.

Curry: The curcumin in tumeric—a spice in curry—lowers stress levels by inhibiting cortisol secretion, says a study from China.

Milk: In a study in the *Archives of Internal Medicine*, women who ate four or more servings of calcium a day had a 30 percent lower risk of PMS symptoms like anxiety and irritability.

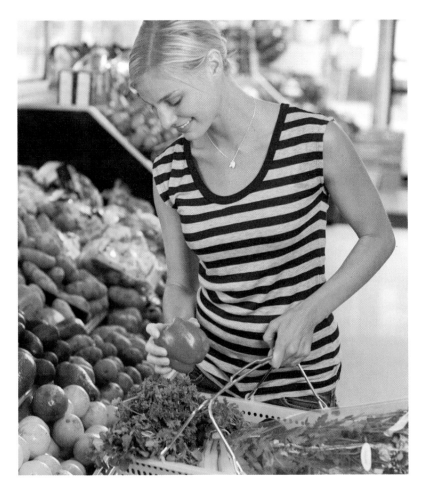

Pistachios: Eating one and a half to three ounces of pistachios daily can lower blood pressure when you're faced with a mentally taxing activity, like taking a test, by relaxing blood vessels, say researchers at Pennsylvania State University.

Red Bell Pepper: Vitamin C, which is abundant in these peppers, lowers stress by limiting cortisol production and stimulates the release of oxytocin, a feel-good chemical. When researchers at the University of Trier in Germany subjected people to the anxiety of public speaking, those who took 3,000 milligrams of C felt calmer, and their blood pressure returned to normal faster than those who skipped the C.

....

Did You Know?
THIS IS THE ULTIMATE STRESS-FIGHTING MEAL: SAUTÉ 2 TEASPOONS CURRY POWDER AND 1 CLOVE MINCED GARLIC IN 2 TEASPOONS COCONUT OIL. ADD ¼ CUP LOWFAT MILK, 12 LARGE SHRIMP, ¼ CUP GREEN PEAS, ¾ CUP COOKED BROWN RICE, 1 CUP SLICED RED BELL PEPPER AND 1 CUP GRATED CARROTS. COOK UNTIL VEGGIES ARE TENDER. TOP WITH 2 TABLESPOONS EACH CHOPPED PISTACHIOS AND RAISINS.

When the Going Gets Tough

Try this 24-hour motivation makeover to recharge any better-body resolution .

First thing in the morning, set several short-term goals for your day. If your big wish is to drop 20 pounds, your mini missions might be: Eat a healthy breakfast; do a three-mile run; choose fruit, not chocolate, for dessert. Smaller goals make your victories more immediate, helping you stay inspired and committed to the process. Many people wind up finding almost as much joy and satisfaction in working toward their accomplishments as they do in achieving them.

To help meet your daily goals, use every mental tool you've got. Often, seeing (and smelling and tasting) is believing. For instance, don't just visualize yourself eating your scrambled eggs on whole-wheat toast. Imagine the aroma, the sound it will make crunching between your teeth, how satisfied you'll feel. Apply all your senses to picture the full spectrum of enjoyment you'll get from doing the thing that moves you closer to your goal.

At the end of the day, reflect on what you've achieved. Then turn your focus to what you can do the next day to keep moving toward the finish line. Write down your ultimate goal and three concrete steps you can take to achieve it. Finish by listing the personal strengths that will enable you to succeed. Finally, claim your goal in the present tense. (Say, "I am 10 pounds thinner," for instance.) Thinking and acting as if you've already reached the mountaintop brings you one step closer to the real deal.

Did You Know?
THE SIDE EFFECTS OF STRESS ARE SERIOUS: ONE IN TWO PEOPLE OVEREAT AND CAN'T SLEEP WHEN THEY'RE STRESSED; AND ONE IN THREE SUFFERS FROM STRESS-INDUCED DEPRESSION. TIME TO FIND CALM, NOW.

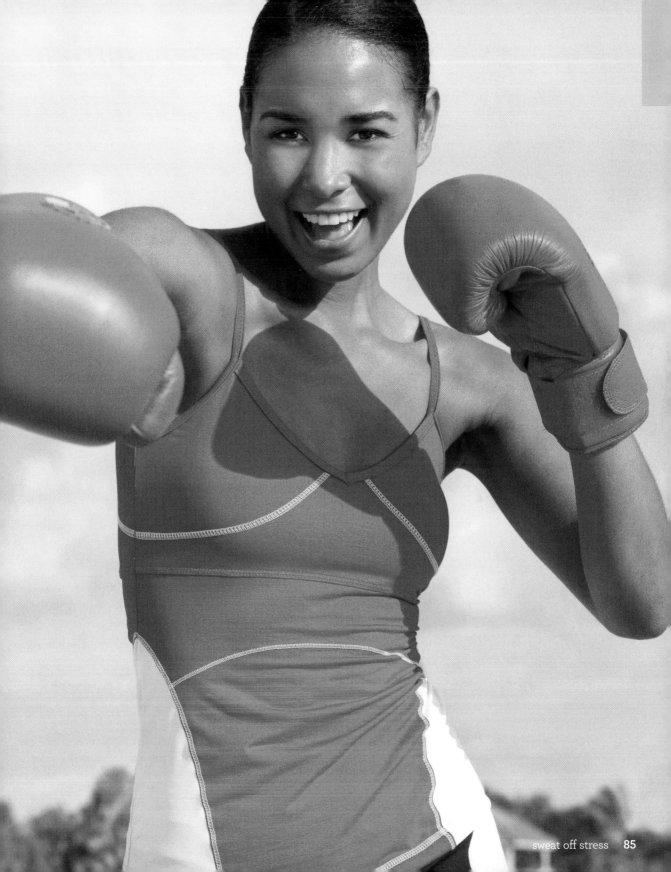

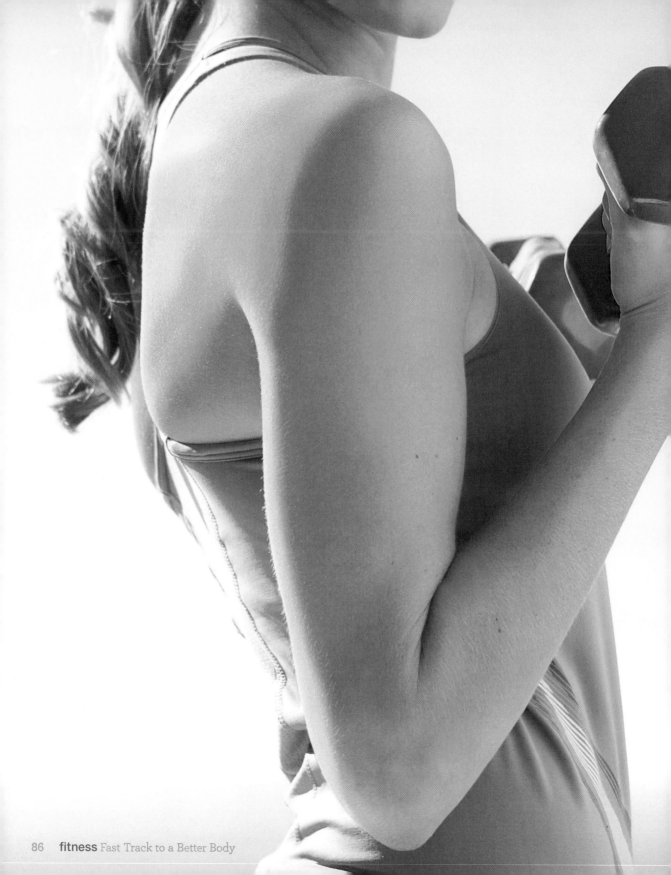

CHAPTER 4

....

strong
sexy
arms

SCULPT YOUR SHOULDERS AND
JIGGLE-PROOF YOUR BICEPS AND TRICEPS
WITH THESE SPEEDY FIRM-UPS.

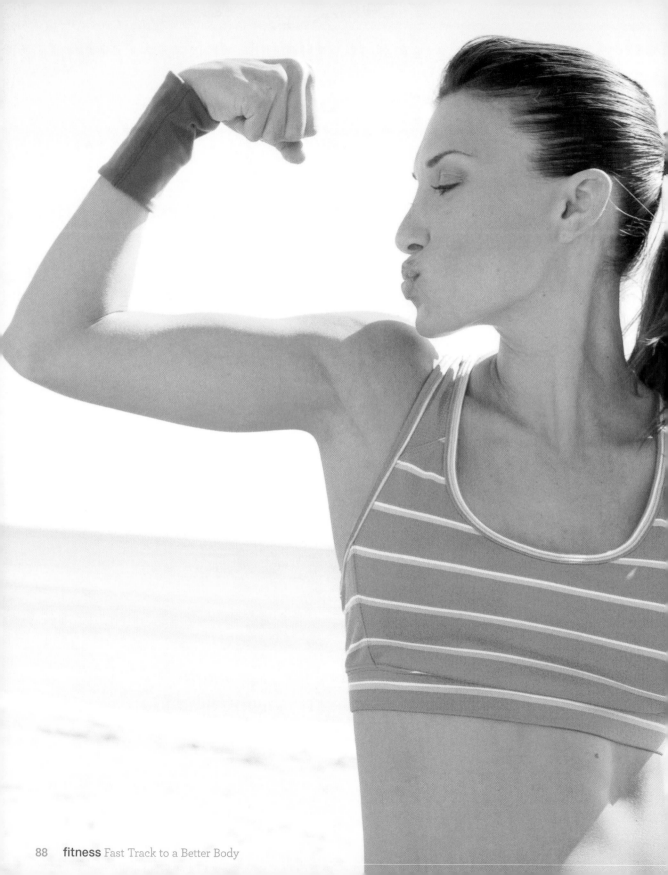

The women who inspire instant arm envy all share one secret: They're not afraid of a little heavy lifting—whether it's a dumbbell or their own body weight. Far too many of us worry about bulking up, so we steer clear of using heavy dumbbells for our arm workouts. Instead, we choose lighter weights and do more repetitions.

That's a good recipe for building your biceps' endurance, but if it's sculpting you're after, never fear adding iron, says Michael Esco, Ph.D., assistant professor of physical education and exercise science at Auburn University at Montgomery in Alabama. Because women have less of the muscle-building hormone testosterone than men do, they can use a heavier weight without developing bulging biceps. In fact, hoisting more pounds is the quickest way to get the sleek, sculpted arms you've been lifting for.

Your best bet when strength training is to start with a weight that will allow you to do 10 reps per set and no more. That means the last two or three reps should feel hard to crank out with good form. Studies have shown that women often pick weights that are too wimpy for the amount of reps they're doing; try a challenging weight to make sure those sets hit the shaping sweet spot.

Week two of your workout, try to do one additional rep. Continue adding one rep per week until you can do 15 reps per set. At that point, switch to a weight that's two pounds heavier and go back

Did You Know? DUMBBELLS GIVE YOU FASTER ARM-SHAPING RESULTS THAN USING JUST YOUR BODY WEIGHT BECAUSE THERE ARE MORE EXERCISES YOU CAN DO WITH THEM, SAYS DR. ESCO. IF YOU'RE TRAVELING, YOU CAN STILL GET IN A GOOD RESISTANCE WORKOUT. PUSH-UPS AND CHAIR DIPS ARE THE BEST WAYS TO USE YOUR BODY WEIGHT TO TONE YOUR ARMS.

to 10 reps. Repeat the same process, working your way up to 15 reps per set. By kicking things up a notch, you'll get better, faster results, Esco says.

Key to Amazing Arms

A quick anatomy lesson: The upper arm is comprised of the biceps in the front and the triceps in the back. The biceps have two muscles (the long and short bicep heads). The triceps have three muscles (the middle, the lateral and the long tricep heads), which make up most of your upper arm. To get defined arms, you need to target both of these muscle groups. Do at least the same amount, if not more, triceps exercises as biceps exercises, Esco suggests. In other words, for every curl you do, you should also do an arm extension exercise, like push-ups.

And don't forget your deltoids, the trio of shoulder muscles—anterior, medial and posterior—that form the coconut shape at the top of each arm. If you're doing a shoulder exercise, such as a lateral raise or a row, you may need to use a different dumbbell than the one you used to do your curls. It takes a bigger load to work your biceps, so you should grab a weight that's on the heavier end for you: maybe 8 to 12 pounds. You'll likely need to lighten your load to 3 or 5 pounds when switching to shoulder moves.

The Tank Top Test

Slip into a tank top and stand in front of a mirror with your arms by your sides. Wishing for more definition? It can be frustrating to feel like you're working hard without seeing results. One reason: Many of us end up doing the same sets of biceps curls again and again. A simple fix is to flip your grip the next time you do them. "After a set of traditional, knuckles-up biceps curls, turn your wrist so that your palms face each other and hinge your forearms out 45 degrees," says Jason Strong, a trainer and manager at Equinox Fitness clubs in New York City. "For the last set, hinge your elbows out to the sides and hold the weights so that your knuckles are facing down."

Now, stand with your side to the mirror. If you're not seeing any sort of divide between your deltoids and upper arm, shoulder exercises may be the TLC your arm needs. Firming flabbiness from the rear view is a job for triceps exercises. The two workout routines in this chapter target all your muscles from every angle to make sure you're covered from top to fingertips.

Show-'Em-Off Secrets

Once they're trim and firm, play up your gorgeous arms with these three simple look-sleek strategies.

Even things out. Smooth rough spots on elbows with an enzyme-based scrub—look for fruit extracts on the label. This ingredient zaps dead cells, revealing newer, healthier skin underneath. Next, apply a rich cream with urea, which not only moisturizes but also dissolves dry layers.

Get a glow safely. Self-tanner will help define the toned muscles in your arms. Apply one layer of tanner with light, sweeping strokes for a subtle natural-looking sheen.

Add flex appeal. For awesome arms in every photo, don't press them into your body. Holding your arms slightly away from your torso will create natural, graceful lines. Want to flaunt your hard work? Lightly flexing arms will help them look more toned.

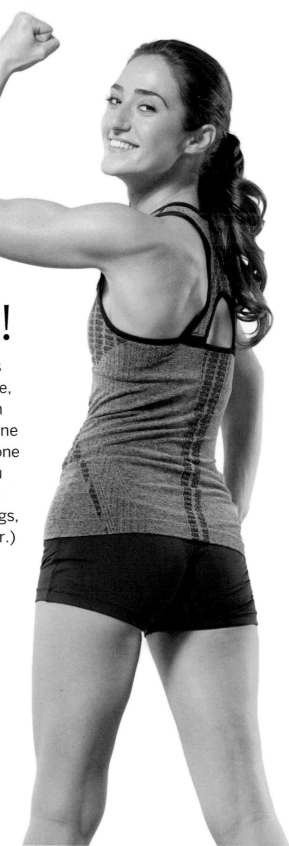

Arm-tastic!

Perform the circuit of exercises on the following five pages twice, resting for 30 seconds between sets. Aim to complete this routine two to three times a week, with one day off between workouts. (You can choose to target a different body part such as your abs or legs, but give arms 48 hours to repair.)

What You'll Need:
A PAIR OF 3- TO 10-POUND DUMBBELLS

21s

Targets biceps

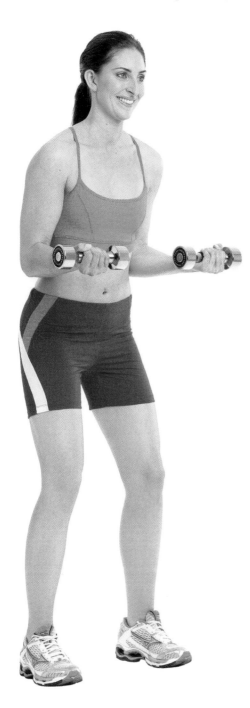

Stand with feet shoulder-width apart, knees slightly bent, holding a dumbbell in each hand, arms by sides, palms facing forward.

Curl dumbbells up to waist level, then lower. Do 7 reps.

After last rep, curl dumbbells from waist up to shoulders; lower to waist. Do 7 reps.

After last rep, lower arms all the way; curl dumbbells up to shoulders and lower. Do 7 reps.

SIDE TRI LIFT

Targets triceps

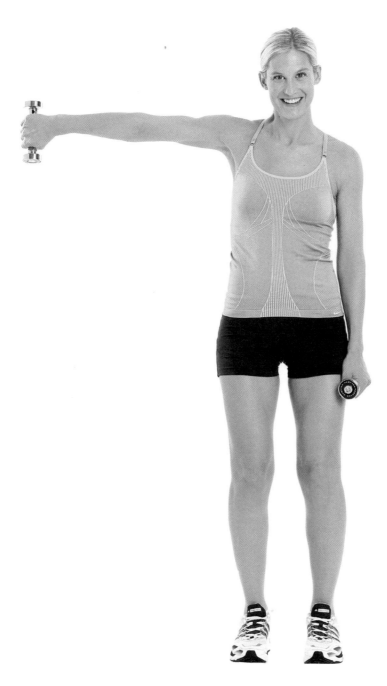

Stand with feet hip-width apart, holding a dumbbell in each hand, arms by sides.

Bend right elbow by side so that right palm is facing shoulder.

Straighten right arm out to side at shoulder level, so that palm faces back.

Lift arm up 2 inches; lower. Bend elbow, bringing hand in front of shoulder again.

Keeping upper arm at shoulder level through-out, extend arm to repeat move.

Do 20 reps; switch arms and repeat.

CURL AND PRESS

Targets shoulders, biceps

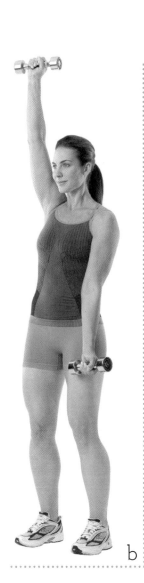

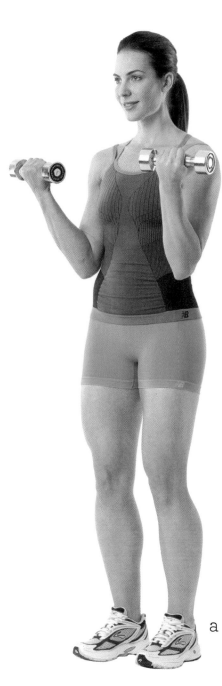

Stand with feet hip-width apart, holding a dumbbell in each hand, palms facing forward.

a. Curl dumbbells up to shoulders.

b. Rotate right palm to face forward and extend right arm overhead while lowering left arm in front of left thigh.

Bend both elbows, bringing dumbbells back in front of shoulders, palms facing body, then reverse the movements, lowering right hand while extending left to complete 1 rep.

Do 10 reps.

JAB, JAB, CROSS

Targets upper back, triceps, legs

Stand with feet shoulder-width apart and staggered (left foot forward, right foot back), knees slightly bent, holding a dumbbell in each hand, arms by sides. Bend elbows, bringing dumbbells in front of shoulders, palms facing in.

a. Throw a double jab: Twist thumb in so palm faces down as you punch left fist forward at shoulder level, then immediately bend elbow to bring dumbbell back in and repeat.

b. Pivot right foot to left and punch right fist forward at shoulder level.

Do 15 reps; switch sides and repeat.

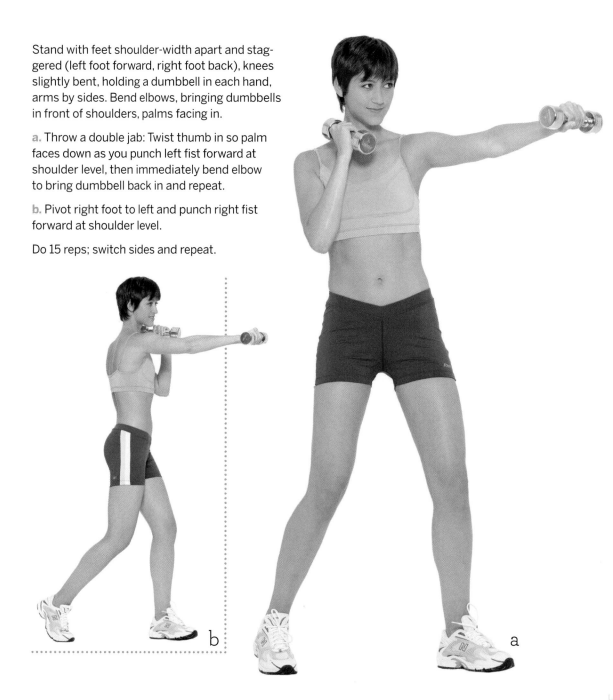

b

a

LOTUS

Targets back, shoulders, abs

Kneel upright on floor with knees under hips, back flat, shoulders down, abs engaged, holding a dumbbell in each hand, arms by sides.

Extend arms out to sides at shoulder level, palms facing up. Exhale and raise arms overhead.

Inhale and slowly lower arms back to shoulder level.

Do 10 reps.

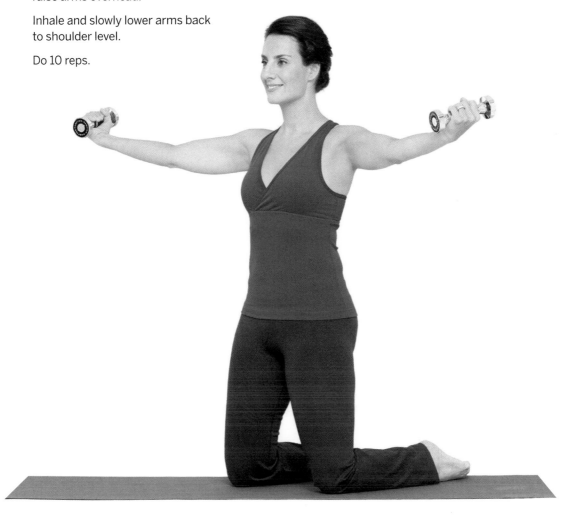

Sleek, Sculpted Arms

Do the following five moves in order, then repeat the circuit once or twice. Complete the workout on nonconsecutive days to give your arm muscles time to rest and repair. Stick with this routine or alternate in the Arm-tastic! workout to firm from fresh angles.

What You'll Need:
A PAIR OF 3- TO 10-POUND DUMBBELLS

FLOATING CURL

Targets upper back, biceps

Stand with feet hip-width apart, knees slightly bent, holding a dumbbell in each hand, arms in front of thighs, palms facing forward.

a. Lift arms straight up to chest level in front of you. Without moving elbows, curl right hand to right shoulder; extend.

b. Repeat with left arm to complete 1 rep.

Do 10 reps, keeping arms lifted throughout.

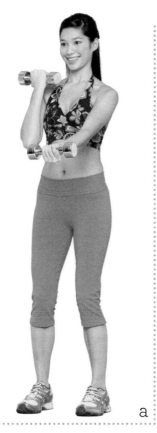

a

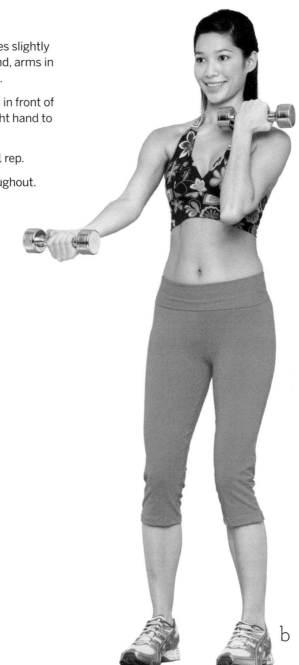

b

SUMO POWER

Targets triceps, butt, inner thighs

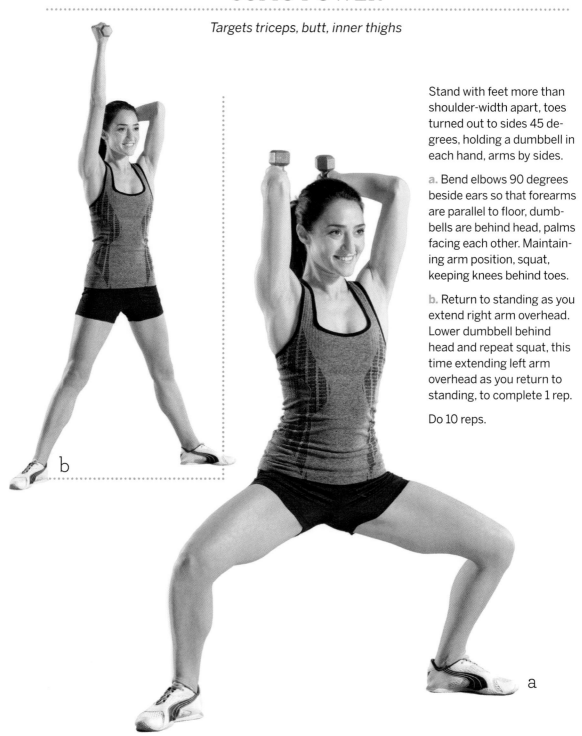

Stand with feet more than shoulder-width apart, toes turned out to sides 45 degrees, holding a dumbbell in each hand, arms by sides.

a. Bend elbows 90 degrees beside ears so that forearms are parallel to floor, dumbbells are behind head, palms facing each other. Maintaining arm position, squat, keeping knees behind toes.

b. Return to standing as you extend right arm overhead. Lower dumbbell behind head and repeat squat, this time extending left arm overhead as you return to standing, to complete 1 rep.

Do 10 reps.

BOXING

Targets shoulders, arms, abs, butt

Stand with feet hip-width apart, holding a dumbbell in each hand, arms by sides. Bend knees and hinge forward from hips until back is parallel to floor. Bend elbows so that they're in line with back.

Keeping abs engaged, exhale as you extend right arm forward, palm facing down, and left arm back, palm facing up.

Pull elbows back in by sides. Switch arms and repeat to complete 1 rep.

Do 4 reps. Roll back up to start.

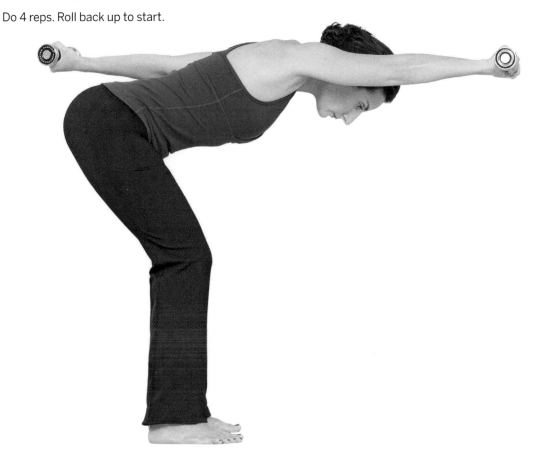

CLEAN AND PRESS

Targets shoulders, back, arms, abs, butt, legs

a. Stand with feet slightly more than shoulder-width apart, knees slightly bent and toes pointed out to sides 45 degrees, holding a dumbbell in right hand. Extend left arm out to side below shoulder level and squat, lowering dumbbell between legs, palm facing body.

b. Thrust up through hips, bending elbow to bring dumbbell in front of shoulder, palm facing left; keep elbow close to body.

Holding dumbbell here, do a half squat, then press right arm straight overhead as you stand up, pressing into heels, to complete 1 rep.

Lower dumbbell to shoulder, then side and repeat.

Do 8 reps. Switch sides, repeat.

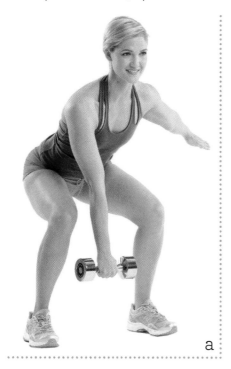

a

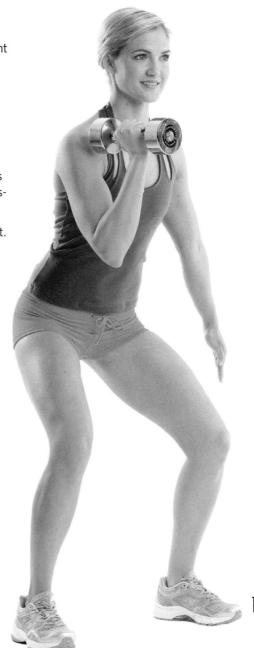

b

KNEE-UP PRESS

Targets shoulders, abs

Sit on floor with knees bent and feet flat on floor, holding a dumbbell in each hand. Bend elbows by sides, bringing dumbbells in front of shoulders, palms facing in.

Keeping shoulders down, lean back slightly and extend arms overhead as you lift feet a few inches off floor, bringing knees toward chest.

Hold position for 1 to 3 counts; lower dumbbells to shoulders and heels to floor to complete 1 rep.

Do 15 reps.

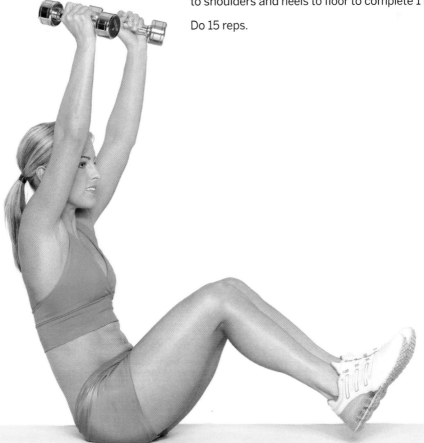

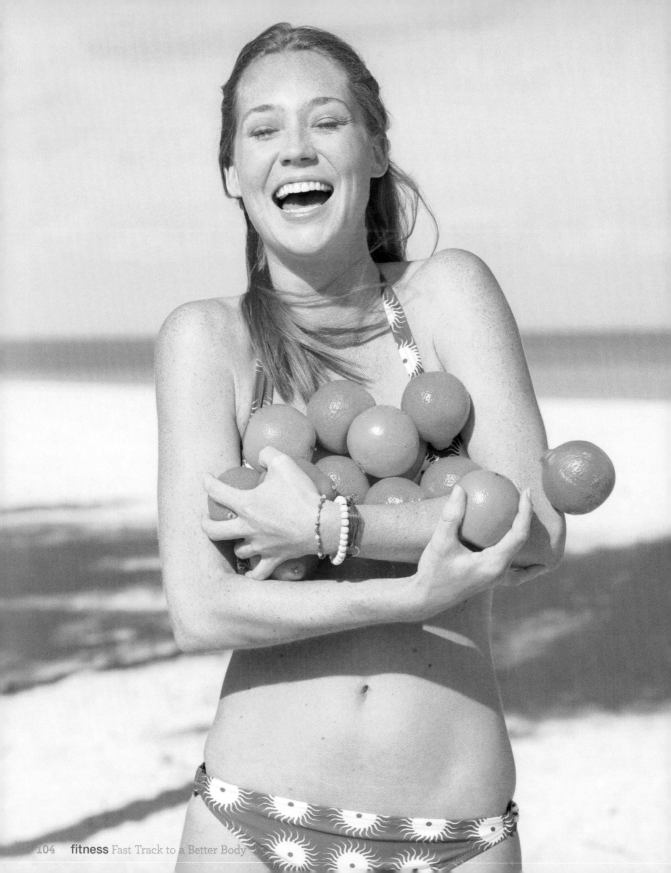

Add Power to Your Diet

To help build leaner, stronger arms, make sure your diet is filled with these nutritional superstars.

Tomato Salsa: This low-cal staple pumps up the flavor of everything from chicken breasts to scrambled eggs. "It's jam-packed with antioxidants, including lycopene, which may reduce the risk of some cancers, and beta-carotene, which may help fight heart disease," says Joan Salge Blake, R.D., an associate clinical professor of nutrition at Boston University.

Eat it up: Beta-carotene and lycopene are more easily absorbed by the body when consumed with a bit of healthy fat, so add some chopped avocado to your salsa-topped chicken. Or add salsa to Low Sodium V8 for extra fiber.

Whole-Wheat Pitas: Give your turkey sandwich a healthy upgrade by swapping the bread for a whole-wheat pita pocket. "Unlike flimsy bread, you can stuff a pita full of vegetables without the sandwich falling apart and still get a healthy dose of whole grains," says Dawn Jackson Blatner, R.D., a FITNESS advisory board member. Just be sure to check the ingredients list for the words "whole wheat." "Enriched wheat flour" means the pita is an imposter.

Eat it up: Go Greek by filling your pita with feta, hummus, diced cucumbers and tomatoes, arugula and black olives. Or put a Mexican spin on your sandwich by adding low-fat refried beans, salsa, avocado and chopped romaine lettuce. Rather have a snack? Make pita chips. Cut a pita into triangles, drizzle with olive oil, add a pinch of salt and bake in the oven at 400 degrees for 10 minutes, or until crispy.

Popcorn: "Because it's super-low in calories, popcorn is the perfect food for those times when you don't want to worry about portion size," says Sharon Richter, R.D., a nutritionist in New York City. And it's loaded with fiber, which is crucial for staying slim. In fact, people who maintain a healthy weight consume an average of 33 percent more fiber daily than those who are overweight.

Eat it up: Using a basic air popper, pop the kernels with a bit of salt and toss with nuts and raisins for a tasty trail mix.

Kale: This leafy green tastes like a slightly sharper version of spinach. Kale is rich in an antioxidant called kaempferol, which Harvard research shows may help lower your chances of developing ovarian cancer by 40 percent. "It's also a great source of iron and folate—which can prevent birth defects—as well as calcium and magnesium, making it a terrific choice for anyone who doesn't eat dairy products," says Dave Grotto, R.D., a FITNESS advisory board member.

Eat it up: Chop the veggie into thin strips and saute in a teaspoon of olive oil with chopped onions and mushrooms for 5 to 10 minutes. Or buy frozen kale to toss into stir-fries, soups, or sauces.

Oranges: Apples get all the glory, but oranges are the unsung heroes of fresh fruit, says Susan Kraus, R.D., a clinical dietitian at Hackensack University Medical Center in New Jersey. "They're very low in calories and a good source of potassium, fiber and folate," Kraus says. Not to mention that a large orange has a day's worth of immunity-boosting vitamin C.

Eat it up: Add orange slices to a spinach salad topped with goat cheese, chopped nuts and some slivered red onion. Or blend 1/2 orange, 1 cup yogurt and 1/2 cup frozen blueberries for a delicious, nutritious smoothie.

Grass-Fed Beef: It has 90 fewer calories and 11 grams less fat per 3.75-ounce serving than corn-fed beef. Plus, "it contains three times more healthy omega-3 fatty acids, which reduce inflammation, improve brain health and lower your risk of heart disease,"

Grotto says. Grass-fed beef is also high in conjugated linoleic acid, a type of polyunsaturated fat that some researchers think may increase weight loss.

Eat it up: Look for meat labeled "100 percent grass-fed." "Organic" doesn't guarantee the cows didn't have grain. Make healthy fajitas: Grill a piece of sirloin, which is relatively low in fat, slice it thinly and serve with grilled veggies, salsa, beans and tortillas.

Vegetable Soup: More than 70 percent of us don't eat the recommended three to five servings of veggies a day. An easy way to help meet your quota is with two cups of vegetable soup. Plus, people who have a bowl before lunch consume 20 percent fewer calories during the meal. The combo of the broth and fiber-rich vegetables increases feelings of fullness, studies show.

Eat it up: Check the sodium content on canned soup—a healthy pick has 480 milligrams or less. Or make your own by sautéing 1 teaspoon olive oil, 1 small chopped onion and 1 teaspoon each minced garlic, dried oregano and dried basil in a pot. Add 2 cups frozen mixed veggies and 4 cups low-sodium vegetable broth, bring to a boil and simmer for 15 minutes. Puree half of the soup for a thicker, richer taste and texture.

Plain Yogurt: "Yogurt contains the perfect ratio of carbohydrates, protein and fat—the carbs give you instant energy, while the protein and fat are released more slowly, keeping you full longer," Kraus says. In a recent study, dieters who consumed three 6-ounce servings of yogurt a day lost 61 percent more body fat overall than those who didn't eat yogurt. The researchers believe that the calcium in dairy increases the activity of enzymes that break down fat cells. Look for yogurt that has at least 20 percent of the RDA.

Eat it up: Mix plain yogurt with a teaspoon of cinnamon or top it with berries for an easy, low-sugar snack. Or use plain Greek yogurt for an extra protein boost in recipes that call for mayo or sour cream, like tuna salad, veggie dip or salad dressings.

Excuse-Proof Your Workout

Pooped? Time-crunched? Just don't feel like it?
Here, your three biggest exercise cop-outs, solved.

I'm too tired. Unless you're incredibly sleep deprived or jet-lagged, there's no reason not to exercise when you're tired, say experts. In fact, working out will rev you up. Researchers at California State University, Long Beach, found that just 10 minutes of brisk walking can give you up to two hours of increased energy. If you need some extra help, try drinking a cup of coffee beforehand. The caffeine jolt can also help improve your exercise performance.

I'm too busy. Many people don't exercise because they feel weighed down with work, but a good sweat session will make you more productive on the job. You'll have less stress, a clearer head and a better perspective. "You can actually get more work done after your workout than before," says Mark Anshel, Ph.D., a performance counselor with LGE Performance Systems, a corporate training center in Orlando, Florida.

I'm not in the mood. If you're feeling out of sorts, a good workout can improve your mood—almost instantly. In a study by the department of exercise science at the University of Georgia in Athens, researchers found that women with high levels of anxiety experienced marked relief after riding a stationary bike for 40 minutes. Many scientists attribute the exercise-induced mood lift to several biochemical changes in the body, including a rush of endorphins to areas of the brain that control emotion and behavior.

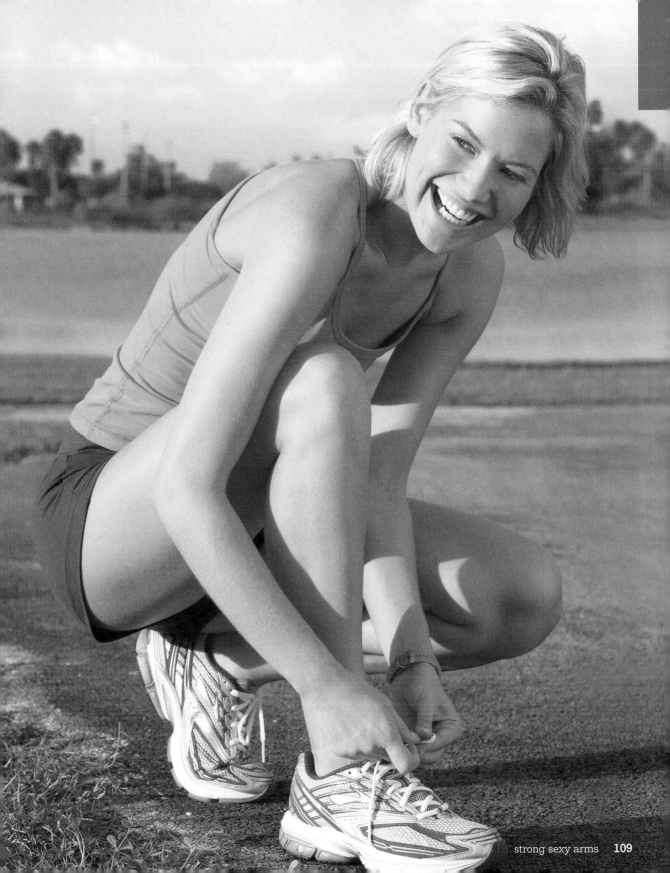

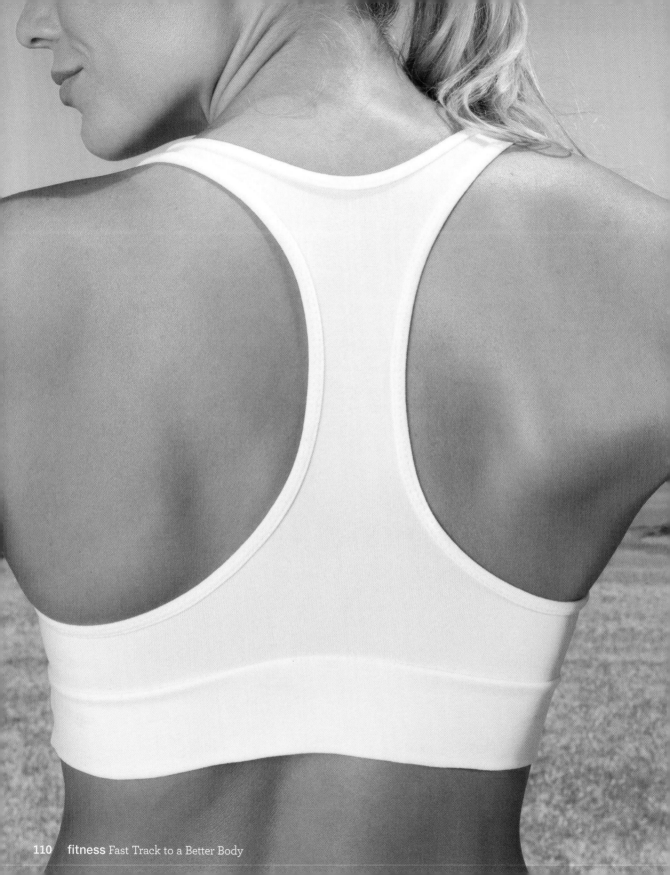

upper body shapers

FOLLOW THESE SUPER-EFFECTIVE WORKOUTS AND EXPERT TIPS TO GET A GORGEOUS CHEST AND BACK.

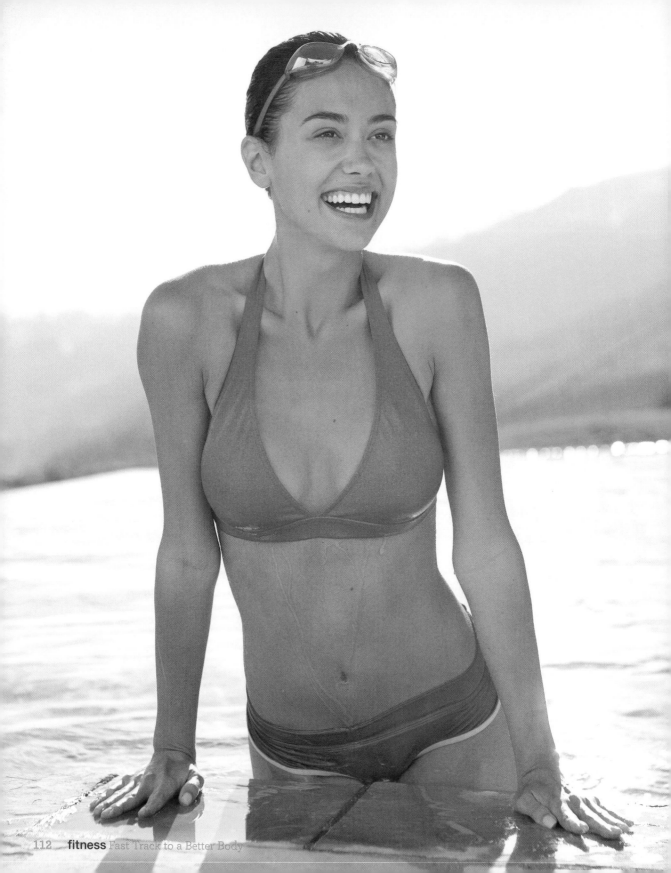

W alk into most gyms, and you'll spot a similar scene: Guys doing a gazillion bench presses and lat pull-downs, and women focusing on their abs and butt. Well, guess what? Experts believe that the scenario should actually be the reverse. "While women's hips and legs tend to be strong, our chest and back muscles are much weaker and less toned naturally than men's," says FITNESS advisory board member Michele Olson, Ph.D., professor of exercise science at Auburn University at Montgomery in Alabama. Not to mention that these often-overlooked zones are vital to getting a great physique. Women have significantly less muscle mass in their upper bodies than men due to genetics, so we need to spend extra time working the muscles there for a balanced figure. And the benefits you get from sculpting your pecs and back don't stop there.

You'll get a bust boost. Seriously: Targeting your chest with push-ups and other resistance moves to reach your deeper chest muscles will give your cleavage a lift. Although your breasts are mostly comprised of connective tissue and fat, you can tone the ligaments underneath. "If you develop these ligaments, as well as the muscle groups in your chest, you'll be able to perk up your breasts, push them out a bit and have natural support that will help prevent sagging," Olson says.

Did You Know?
STRONG CHEST AND BACK MUSCLES STABILIZE YOU DURING WORKOUTS LIKE RUNNING, BIKING, SWIMMING AND LIFTING WEIGHTS, AND KEEP YOU FROM GETTING INJURED.

You'll prevent backaches. Your back muscles are designed to keep the spine straight and aligned. Strengthen them with the right exercises, experts say, and you could skip the nagging back soreness that four out of five women experience at some point in their lives. Use the moves from this chapter—along with the core strengtheners in Chapter 6—for a healthy, strong and pain-free back.

You'll look slimmer. To lessen your love handles and cinch your waist, don't overlook lower back moves. "Think of your body as a cylinder," Olson says. "If you want a smaller waistline, you have to attack it from 360 degrees—the front, the side and the back." Not only do back moves frequently get shortchanged for crunches, but because we stay seated for so many hours—at work, in the car, on the couch—these muscles get stretched and can quickly turn to mush. The stronger your back muscles, the straighter you'll stand, and the trimmer your whole torso will look.

To reap all these better-body rewards and more, your mission is to firm your back and chest muscles so that they're equally balanced. The key is to do the same amount of push exercises (like chest presses) and pull moves (like bent-over rows) each time you strength-train, as in the two workouts in this chapter.

TLC for Your Top Half

When you're following a workout regimen, the drill is sweat, shower, repeat. Turns out, the skin on your chest and back take more of a beating than other body parts do thanks to this get-clean routine. Before you set out on your upper body transformation, keep these save-your-skin secrets in mind.

Rejuvenate dry skin. It takes eight hours for skin to naturally replenish the moisture it loses from a shower, according to research by beauty manufacturer Dove. And your chest, back and torso can be left drier than your lower half because hot water hits the skin there first, says Elissa Lunder, M.D., a dermatologist in Wellesley,

Q: **WHAT'S THE BEST WAY TO TEST A SPORTS BRA BEFORE I BUY IT?**

A: First, consider the intensity of your typical workout, says Alma Adrovic, product designer for global women's training at Nike. (Light activities include yoga and strength training; medium-impact is cycling or brisk walking; and high-impact is running.) Choose several bras in the proper intensity category and try them on. Check the chest band—it should be tight enough for you to comfortably slip one finger underneath it. Next, bend forward. The bra's cups should provide enough coverage and support so that your breasts stay in place. Finally, the straps should be snug, but not digging into your skin. Test them by raising your arms above your head. If the chest band of the bra moves up, the straps are too tight.

Massachusetts, and a FITNESS advisory board member. To protect your skin, use warm, not hot, water plus a body scrub to lift dead skin, and call it quits after 10 minutes. Immediately post-shower, apply body lotion or cream on damp skin. "Like a wet sponge, damp skin absorbs moisture more readily than dry," says Annet King of cosmetic company Dermalogica. Intensify your lotion's power by mixing it with a teaspoon of body oil.

Beat breakouts. Sweat often pools on your décolletage as you exercise. After you work out, apply a layer of clay-infused cleanser (look for the ingredient kaolin on the label) to the area and rinse. The minerals work with shower steam to draw out dirt and excess oil. Wipe an astringent pad over the upper back post-workout to prevent pimples and blackheads.

Erase stubborn spots. Blame the sun for those blotches on your chest, a common problem for outdoor exercisers. "Many women don't put sunblock on that area,"says Ranella Hirsch, M.D., a dermatologist in Cambridge, Massachusetts. Since the skin on your chest is less sensitive than your face, you can use a peel with glycolic acid, which gently strips away some pigment. To prevent marks in the future, wear a broad-spectrum SPF 30 sunscreen daily.

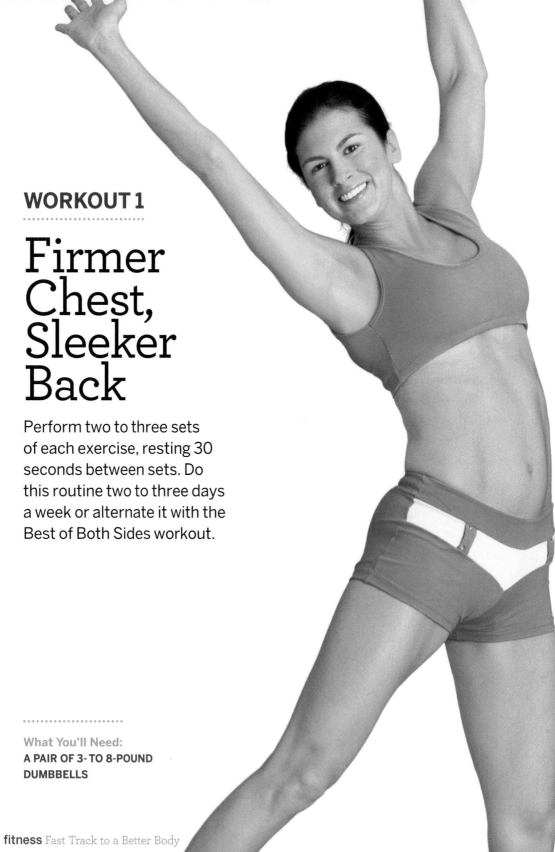

Firmer Chest, Sleeker Back

Perform two to three sets
of each exercise, resting 30
seconds between sets. Do
this routine two to three days
a week or alternate it with the
Best of Both Sides workout.

What You'll Need:
**A PAIR OF 3- TO 8-POUND
DUMBBELLS**

GIMME A Y! GIMME A T!

Targets shoulders, upper back, abs, butt, legs

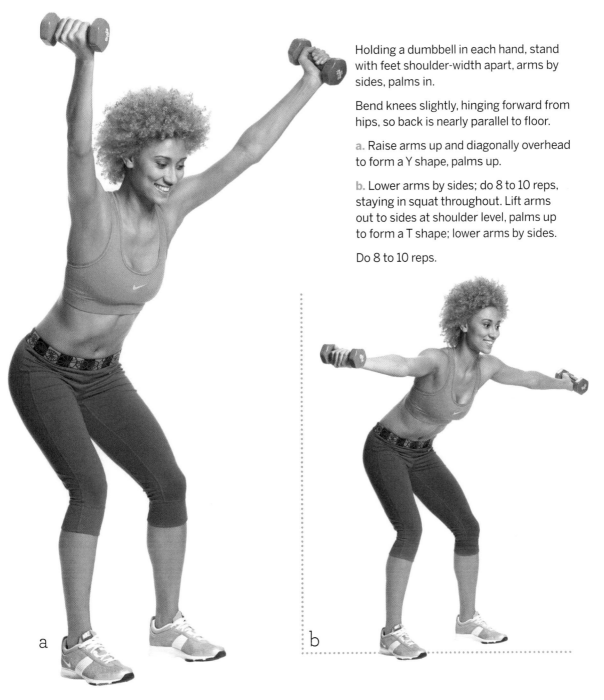

Holding a dumbbell in each hand, stand with feet shoulder-width apart, arms by sides, palms in.

Bend knees slightly, hinging forward from hips, so back is nearly parallel to floor.

a. Raise arms up and diagonally overhead to form a Y shape, palms up.

b. Lower arms by sides; do 8 to 10 reps, staying in squat throughout. Lift arms out to sides at shoulder level, palms up to form a T shape; lower arms by sides.

Do 8 to 10 reps.

a

b

DOUBLE-LIFT PUSH-UP

Targets shoulders, upper back, chest, abs, obliques

Holding a dumbbell in each hand, get into full push-up position (balancing on hands and toes so body is parallel with floor), hands under shoulders, palms in.

a. Keeping abs engaged, bend elbows to lower chest toward floor.

b. Extend arms again to do a push-up, then pull right elbow toward ceiling, bringing dumbbell next to ribs while keeping left arm straight. Hold for 1 count and lower right arm; repeat with left arm to complete 1 rep.

Do 5 reps.

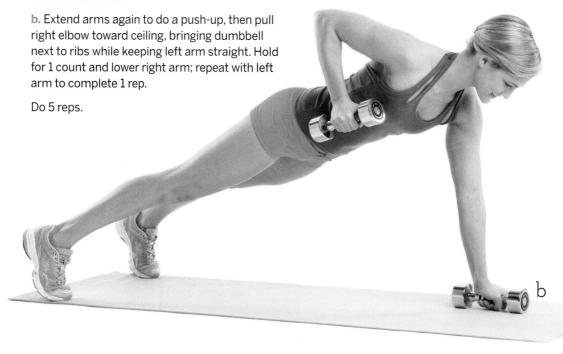

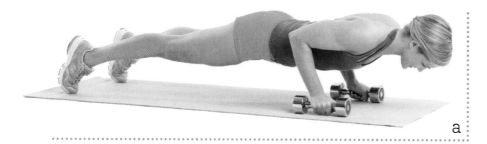

BACK TOUCH

Targets back, shoulders, biceps

Holding a dumbbell in each hand, stand with feet hip-width apart, arms by sides. Extend arms diagonally out to sides so they're about one foot behind you, palms down.

a. Bend left elbow and touch back with dumbbell; extend.

b. Switch arms and repeat to complete 1 rep.

Do 15 reps.

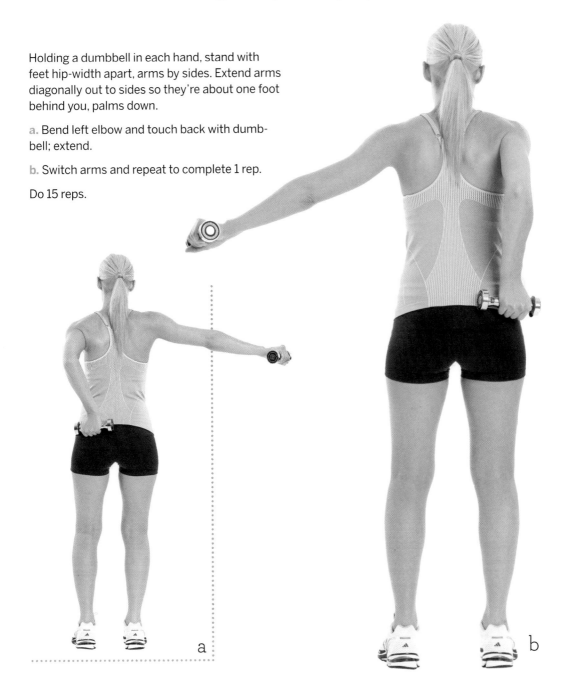

a

b

CHEST FLYE BICYCLE

Targets chest, abs

Holding a dumbbell in each hand, lie faceup on floor with knees bent 90 degrees over hips, arms extended directly above chest, palms in.

a. Keeping right knee bent, straighten left leg toward floor.

b. Lower arms out to sides with elbows slightly bent. Hold for 1 count, then return to start.

Do 10 reps; switch legs and repeat.

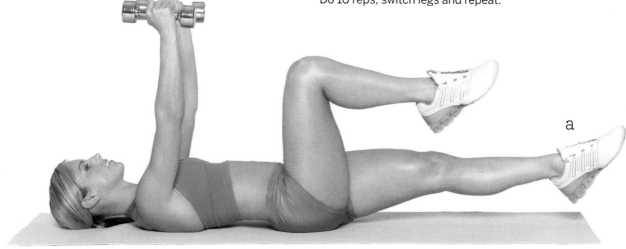

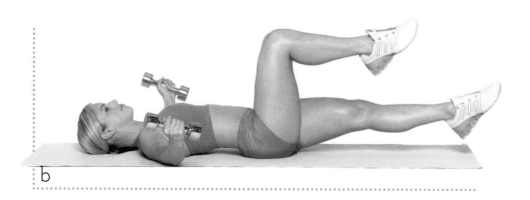

HAMSTRING CURL, BACK EXTENSION

Targets shoulders, back, hamstrings

a. Holding a dumbbell in each hand, lie facedown on floor with legs together, arms extended overhead, palms down. Lift arms and head a few inches off floor, keeping head in line with spine.

b. Bend knees, bringing feet toward butt, while bending elbows down by sides, pulling dumbbells down to shoulder level. Squeeze shoulder blades together and release, extending arms and legs.

Do 10 reps, keeping arms and head lifted throughout.

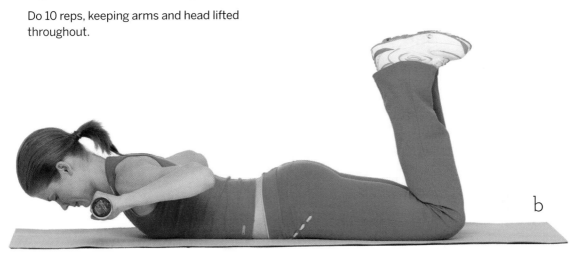

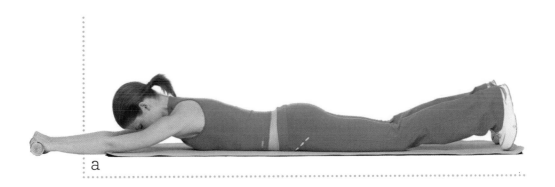

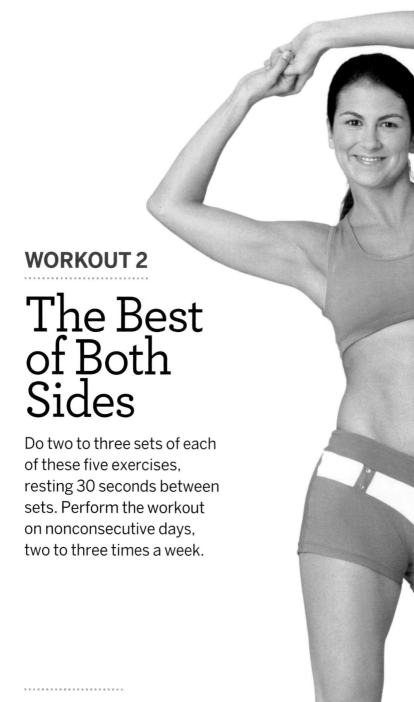

The Best of Both Sides

Do two to three sets of each of these five exercises, resting 30 seconds between sets. Perform the workout on nonconsecutive days, two to three times a week.

What You'll Need:
A PAIR OF 3- TO 8-POUND DUMBBELLS AND A STABILITY BALL

PLANK WALKUP

Targets arms, abs, chest, back, glutes

a. Get into plank position, balancing on floor on forearms and toes.

b. Keeping back straight, abs engaged and legs together, extend right arm, then left to press into full push-up position.

Gently "walk" hands back down to plank, lowering onto right forearm, then left forearm.

Do 5 reps without lowering body to floor.

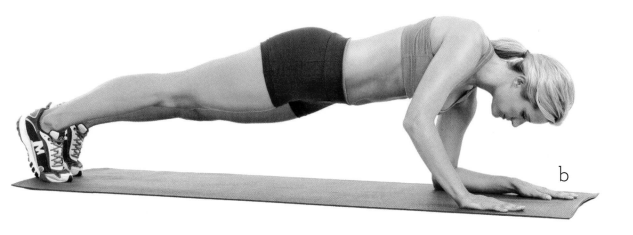

b

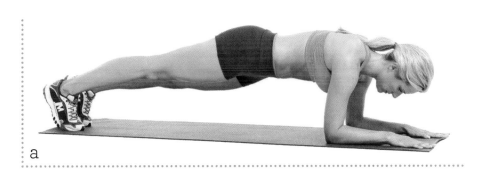

a

WIDE-STANCE DEADLIFT

Targets lower back, butt, legs

Holding a dumbbell in each hand, stand with feet more than shoulder-width apart, toes pointed out 45 degrees, arms in front of thighs, palms in.

Keeping back straight and knees slightly bent, hinge forward from hips as you lower dumbbells to shin level. Return to start.

Do 12 reps.

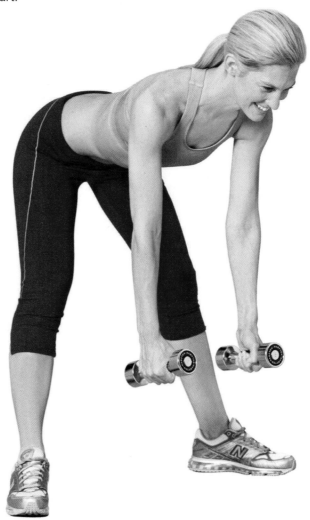

BRIDGE PRESS PLUS

Targets chest, arms, abs, butt

Holding a dumbbell in each hand, lie faceup on floor with knees bent and feet flat, arms by sides. Bend elbows 90 degrees so that forearms are perpendicular to floor, upper arms still on floor, palms facing each other.

a. Lift hips slowly off floor, forming a straight line from knees to shoulders, and maintain bridge position throughout. Then press dumbbells straight up toward ceiling, above shoulders.

b. Keeping upper arms still, bend elbows 90 degrees to lower dumbbells behind you so that forearms are parallel to floor.

Extend arms toward ceiling, then lower elbows to floor to complete 1 rep.

Do 12 reps.

REVERSE FLYE

Targets shoulders, back

Holding a dumbbell in each hand, stand with feet shoulder-width apart, arms by sides, palms in.

Keeping back flat and abs engaged, hinge forward from hips and lift arms out to sides at shoulder level, keeping elbows slightly bent; lower.

Do 12 reps, maintaining bent-over position throughout.

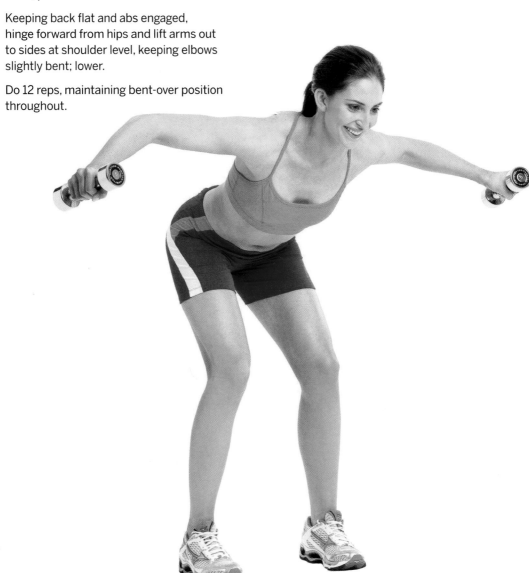

RAINBOW FLYE

Targets shoulders, chest, arms, abs

Holding a dumbbell in each hand, lie faceup on a stability ball with upper back resting on ball, knees bent 90 degrees and feet flat, so torso is parallel to floor.

Extend arms out to sides at shoulder level, keeping elbows slightly bent, palms facing up.

Raise arms toward ceiling, rotating wrists as you lift so palms face forward and ends of dumbbells meet in center directly above chest. Lower arms back out to sides.

Do 12 reps.

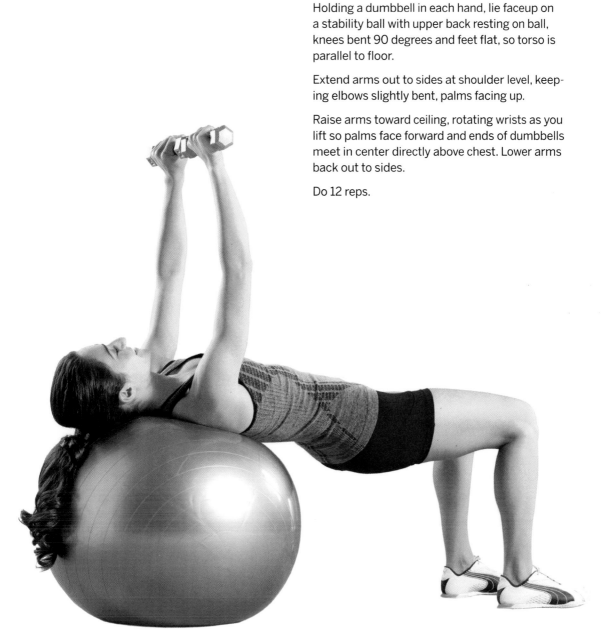

Pain-Proof Your Back

Simple and effective strategies to stay ache-free

Shift into neutral. Your spine is meant to be in a neutral position—with a moderate inward curve in the lower back and a moderate outward curve in the upper back. "Teach" it how to stay put: Stand with your back, shoulders and heels against a wall and place one hand behind your back, feeling the slight curve in your spine. Do this posture check a few times a day to set your back in neutral.

Sit properly. Even the simple act of sitting can put a great deal of stress on the lower spine. To reduce this pressure, keep your hips and knees flexed at a 90-degree angle and sit up tall. Placing the balls of your feet about shoulder-width apart on a one- or two-inch footrest will help prevent you from slouching, says Gayle Jasinski, a chiropractor with the Texas Back Institute in Plano. If you have a desk job, take a break every half hour: Stand, stretch or walk around for one or two minutes to help "reset" your posture when you sit. If you can't leave your workspace, take phone calls standing up.

Lighten up. Do you really need to haul around four magazines, your laptop, a liter of water, a cell phone and a pair of shoes every time you leave the house? Women who carry more than five to 10 pounds on one shoulder risk getting aches in their upper back from the weight, says Jasinski. Reduce your burden by determining what's critical to carry, then splitting it into two relatively even loads and carrying a bag on each shoulder. Better yet, wear a backpack (slipped over both shoulders) to transfer much of the weight onto your stronger upper-back muscles.

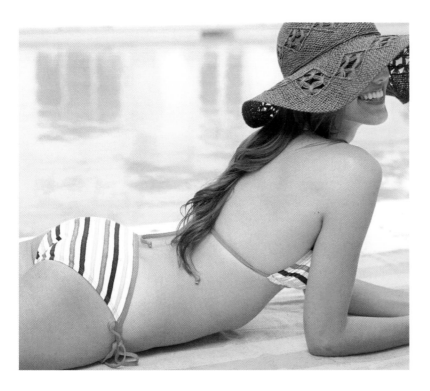

Do the single-leg lift. When you bend over to pick up light objects (like a stray shoe or a toy), lift one leg a couple of inches behind you and contract your abs for a few seconds, says Stuart McGill, Ph.D., a professor of spine biomechanics at the University of Waterloo in Canada. Do this several times a day and you'll quickly feel your back and core muscles grow stronger. To lift heavier objects, such as a basket of laundry, it's best to squat first, holding the object close to your body to avoid overextending your back. And remember to tighten your abs in this position for added back protection.

Warm up your spine. Whether you're about to step onto the tennis court or you're waiting for an exercise class to begin, take two minutes to reduce the stiffness of your back by warming up with a cat/cow exercise. Start on all fours on the floor, then slowly round your back like a cat; gently release, arching slightly and keeping abs tight throughout. For the safest and most effective stretch, think about gradually moving the spine rather than jerking into the poses.

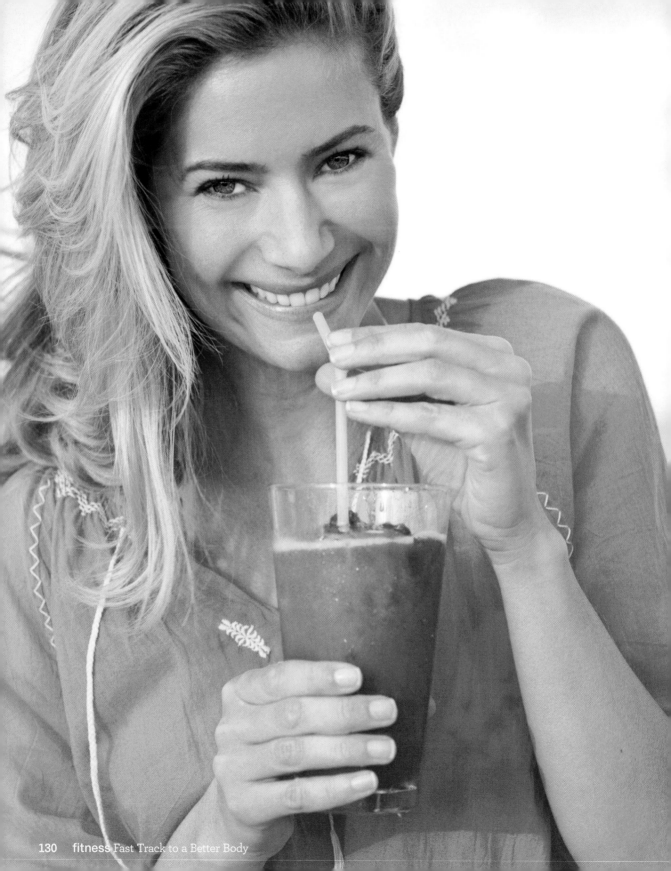

Heart-Healthy Eats

These 11 ingredients will lower your blood pressure and your cholesterol to help keep your ticker in top shape.

Blueberries: Bursting with antioxidants, these nutritional powerhouses help fight inflammation and lower bad LDL cholesterol and blood sugar.

Olive and Canola Oil: These are high in heart-smart monounsaturated fats and lower in unhealthy saturated fat than other oils.

Cinnamon: Studies show that this spice lowers LDL cholesterol and raises good HDL cholesterol.

Oatmeal: The breakfast favorite is a great source of soluble fiber. And it's full of heart-friendly B vitamins.

Nuts: Almonds and walnuts are packed with heart helpers, like omega-3 fatty acids, potassium and vitamin E.

Salmon: The omega-3s in this fish help reduce bad cholesterol and make your blood flow smoothly, lessening the chance of clotting.

Flaxseeds: They're rich in alpha-linolenic acid, a fatty acid that may help regulate blood pressure, blood fat and inflammation. Sprinkle some on your salad, cereal or yogurt cup.

Spinach: This dark leafy green is loaded with B vitamins and antioxidants that help fight heart disease, plus magnesium to help lower blood pressure.

Red Wine and Grape Juice: These beverages are brimming with antioxidants to help strengthen your heart.

Legumes: Beans and lentils are chock-full of soluble fiber, which has been shown to help lower cholesterol.

White Potatoes: The notoriously diet-busting starch can actually be a part of a healthy diet, due to high amounts of vitamin B6, which helps prevent heart disease.

Did You Know? A MORNING MEAL HELPS REGULATE BLOOD SUGAR AND CHOLESTEROL, WHICH CAN REDUCE YOUR RISK OF HEART DISEASE. TRY A VEGGIE OMELET WITH A WHOLE-GRAIN ENGLISH MUFFIN.

Make Over Your Mojo

These motivation boosters will get you back on track, no matter what your better-body goal.

Roadblock: Last month, you were gung-ho about your new workout routine. Now you're just not feeling it. It's a battle to get psyched about exercise.

Clear the hurdle: Many people think we need to motivate before we take action, but the opposite is also true—by acting, we can motivate ourselves. If you can force yourself to just get up and get moving, experts say, within minutes it will become easier and your attitude will change.

Roadblock: It's 3 p.m. and your sugar craving is calling. Loudly.

Clear the hurdle: It's not about the candy bar. It's about what's going on in your head. Soothing your emotions with food is much easier than facing them head-on. The trick is to recognize the frenzied thought pattern that beckons you toward the fridge or the vending machine—and force your mind to slow down. Stop, take a deep breath and go for a walk instead.

Roadblock: You constantly compare your body to others at the gym—and find yourself coming up short.

Clear the hurdle: Turn envy into admiration and an incentive to improve. See someone with great abs? Take it as a challenge to work harder on your own core. But don't lose sight of why you're at the gym in the first place. You want to get fit, not win the best booty contest. Concentrate on working out to shape up and get stronger—and to feel better overall.

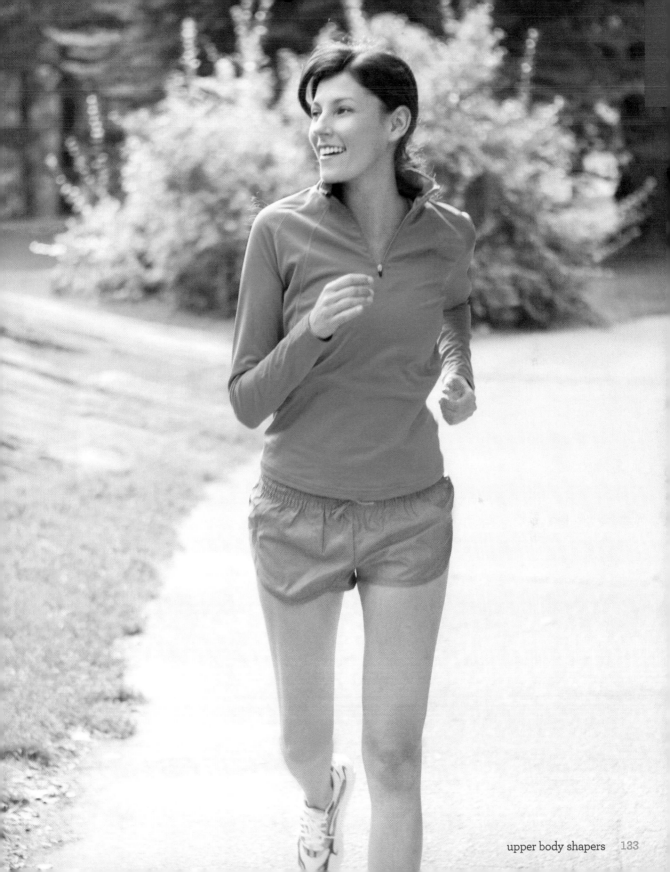

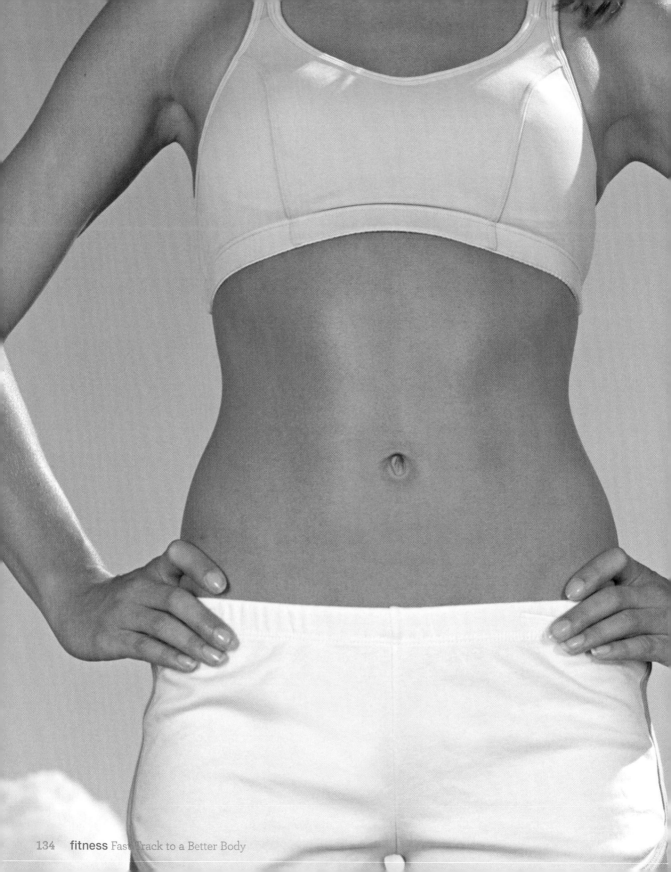

CHAPTER 6

flat abs fast

CONSIDER THIS YOUR TRIMMER-BELLY BLUEPRINT, INCLUDING ALL THE MOVES, MEALS AND MOTIVATION YOU NEED.

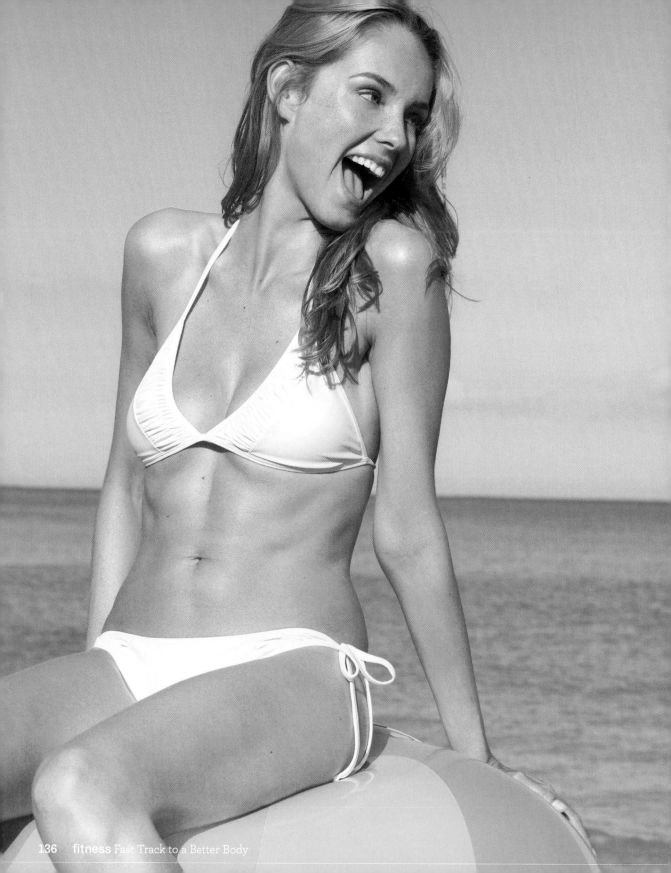

The days of doing hundreds of sit-ups in pursuit of a flat belly are over. Science has since found an upgrade for the common crunch, and the two breakthrough routines in this chapter will prove it to you.

Your midsection is made up of more muscles than meet the mirror. While moves like sit-ups and crunches can strengthen the front "six-pack" muscle known as the rectus abdominis, that's only part of the story. The rectus is often the center of attention for exercisers because it's the abdominal muscle that's closest to the surface. Its primary function is to bend your spine forward, so sit-ups became the top pick for working it into washboard shape.

Although you may have heard of upper versus lower abs, the rectus abdominis is all one sheath of muscle. So even though you might feel a certain exercise more in the upper half, the lower half is also engaged, and vice versa. Where you feel the effort most depends on the move's anchor point. For example, leg lifts engage more of the lower area because your upper body is against the floor.

However, there is another major player that makes up your abdominals. The deepest layer of abdominal muscle is called the transverse abdominis. It runs horizontally across your midsection like a corset, stabilizing your trunk and core. Work this muscle with moves like planks and you'll really hit the waist-cinching sweet spot.

Did You Know? LIKE OTHER MUSCLES, YOUR ABS RESPOND BEST TO INTENSE TRAINING EVERY OTHER DAY, WITH A DAY OFF IN BE- TWEEN TO ALLOW THE MUSCLES TO RECOVER AND GROW STRONGER.

Rounding out your core crew are the obliques—internal and external—the muscles that run on a diagonal up the sides of your midsection from your pelvis to the bottom of your rib cage. You'll feel these muscles activated when you do rotating movements like trunk twists.

Before you flip to the workouts in this chapter, let's get back to those crunches. Are they worth the sweat? Yes, but if you're doing more than three sets of 15, you're wasting your time, says FITNESS advisory board member Michele Olson, Ph.D., a professor of exercise science at Auburn University at Montgomery in Alabama. "Extra crunches aren't going to cinch your waistline," says Olson. "You're working the rectus abdominis, but it's the other three deeper muscles that give you a leaner look by helping you with your posture."

The bottom line is that to truly tone your middle, you need to do a mix of ab moves in varying positions. And to get the most visible results from these supershapers, you need to pair them with the right combination of diet and calorie-burning cardio exercise.

The Truth About Ab Flab

It seems like every time you put on a pound or two, the extra weight goes straight to your waist. Sure, you can suck it in to zip it up, but carrying around that pudge can be a major bummer.

To fight abdominal fat effectively, it helps to understand exactly what you're targeting. Subcutaneous fat is the stuff right under your skin. It's commonly found in your abdomen and also your butt and thighs.

But the true troublemaker is visceral, or "toxic," fat, found deep in your abdomen below your ab muscles. Visceral fat is so dangerous because it surrounds your organs and secretes toxic hormones, which contribute to the thickening of the walls of coronary blood vessels, increasing your chances of having a heart attack. Study after study shows that belly fat increases your risk of heart disease and high blood pressure, among other health woes. Not only that, women whose waists are bigger than 35 inches are more than twice as likely to die of heart disease than women whose middles measure less than 28 inches, according to research from the National Institutes of Health. And a waist that's more than 32 inches increases your risk of diabetes, experts say.

Now for the good news: Before menopause, women lose weight far more easily from their bellies than from their thighs or buttocks. One of the most effective ways to decrease flab around your middle is to sweat it off. And while it's not possible to spot -reduce, some research suggests that abdominal fat may be more responsive to exercise than fat in other areas.

Cutting calories is also key to maximizing your middle-whittling efforts. The trick is finding that perfect mix of meals to get the job done fastest. The Flat Abs Diet in this chapter is a well-balanced way to lose 5 pounds in four weeks. The twist: It's got ingredients built into it that have been proven to specifically help you drop abdominal fat. It's true—the foods you choose can determine where you lose, and this diet has a bull's-eye on your abs.

Whether you measure your success by your scale or your waistband, follow the workouts and other to-do's on these pages and you'll see visible results in a month.

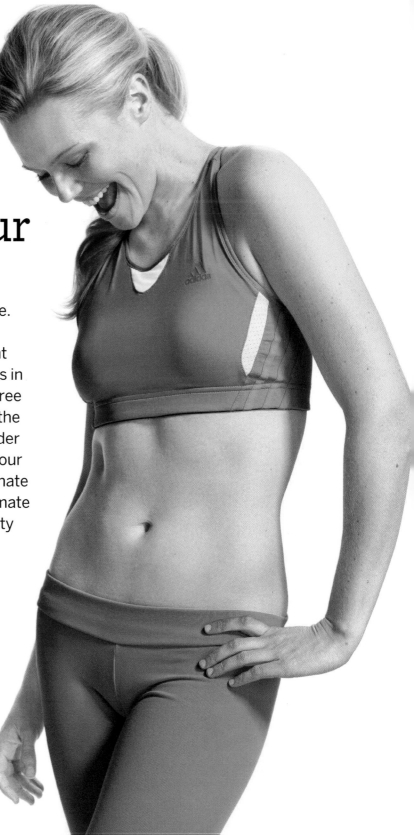

WORKOUT 1

Slim Your Center

The muffin top stops here. You won't need anything but your own body weight to perform the five moves in this routine. Do two to three sets of each exercise on the following pages in the order shown. Aim for three to four sessions a week, or alternate this routine with the Ultimate Tummy Trimmers stability ball workout.

STANDING SIDE CRUNCH

Targets abs, obliques, butt

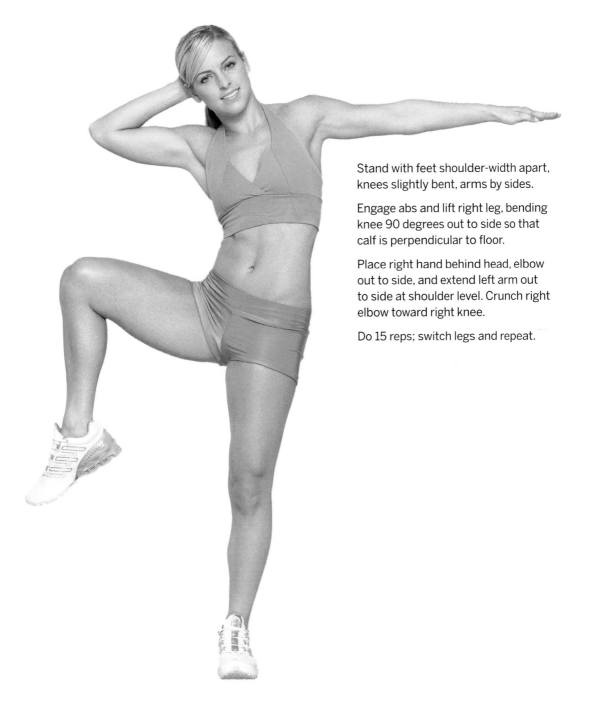

Stand with feet shoulder-width apart, knees slightly bent, arms by sides.

Engage abs and lift right leg, bending knee 90 degrees out to side so that calf is perpendicular to floor.

Place right hand behind head, elbow out to side, and extend left arm out to side at shoulder level. Crunch right elbow toward right knee.

Do 15 reps; switch legs and repeat.

AERIAL PLIÉ

Targets abs, legs

Sit on floor with legs extended, heels together, toes pointed out to sides.

a. Place hands behind head, elbows out to sides. Lift legs about 2 feet, lean back 45 degrees, abs engaged.

b. Flex feet, heels together, and bend knees into chest (like a frog); extend legs, keeping back tall and heels together.

Do 15 reps.

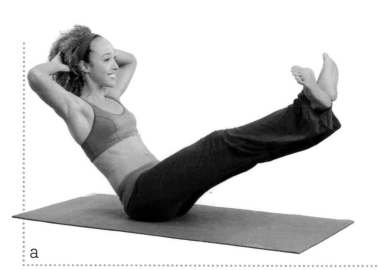

a

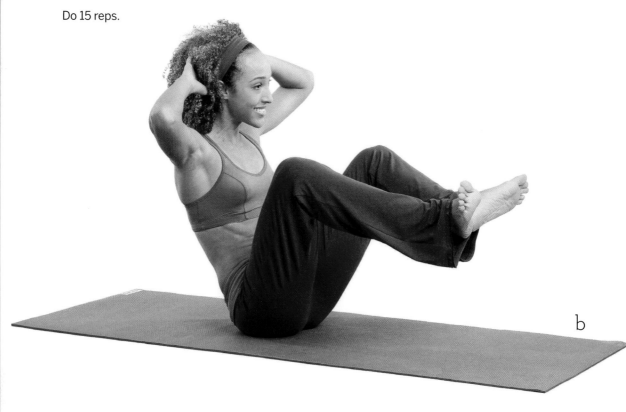

b

DOUBLE CROSS

Targets back, abs, obliques, shoulders

Start in full push-up position (balancing on hands and toes so body is parallel to floor) with feet slightly more than shoulder-width apart.

Lift left leg up, cross it over and to right of right leg, then tap left toes on floor. Return to start.

Lift right leg up, cross it over and to left of left leg, then tap right toes on floor. Return to start to complete 1 rep.

Do 8 reps.

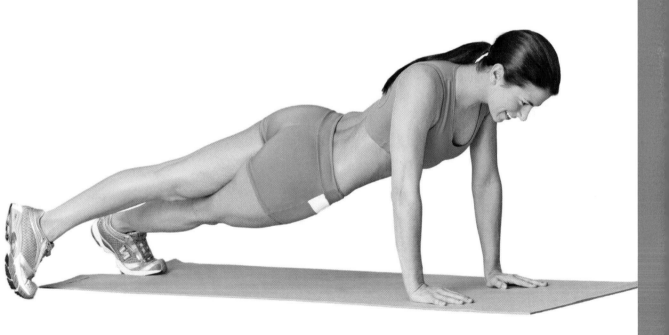

PIKE AND EXTEND

Targets abs, legs

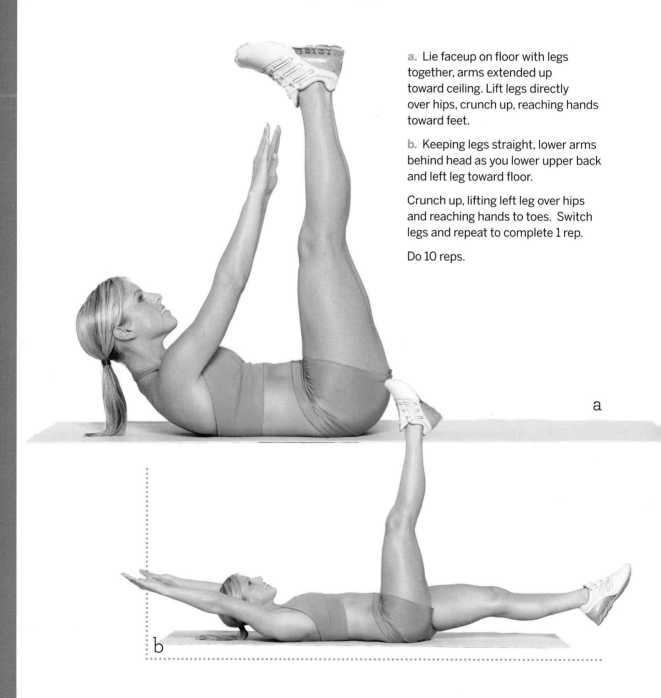

a. Lie faceup on floor with legs together, arms extended up toward ceiling. Lift legs directly over hips, crunch up, reaching hands toward feet.

b. Keeping legs straight, lower arms behind head as you lower upper back and left leg toward floor.

Crunch up, lifting left leg over hips and reaching hands to toes. Switch legs and repeat to complete 1 rep.

Do 10 reps.

a

b

WINDSHIELD WIPER

Targets abs, obliques

a. Lie faceup on floor with arms extended diagonally out to sides just below shoulder level, palms down, legs together. Lift legs directly over hips.

b. Engage abs and slowly lower legs together toward right as far as you can while maintaining good form (lower so right toes touch floor, if you can).

Lift legs back to start; drop legs to left and return to start to complete 1 rep.

Do 8 reps.

b

a

Ultimate Tummy Trimmers

Using a stability ball has been scientifically proven to turn up the firming power of ab exercises otherwise performed on the floor. Do each move in order, repeating the circuit to complete two to three sets. Try to do three to four sessions a week.

What You'll Need:
A STABILITY BALL
To find one that's right for your height, follow this guide:

Under 5' – 5'3"	45 cm ball
5'3 – 5'7"	55 cm ball
Over 5'7"	65 cm ball

BEACH BALLET

Targets shoulders, abs, butt, quads

Stand with feet hip-width apart, holding a stability ball with arms extended at shoulder level in front of you.

a. Keeping abs engaged, lift right foot off floor and bring bent right knee up to hip level in front of you.

b. Bend left knee slightly and press right heel back so that right leg extends behind you as you lift ball diagonally overhead and lean forward, forming a straight line.

Straighten body as you bend right knee in front of you and lower ball to shoulder level.

Do 10 reps. Switch sides; repeat.

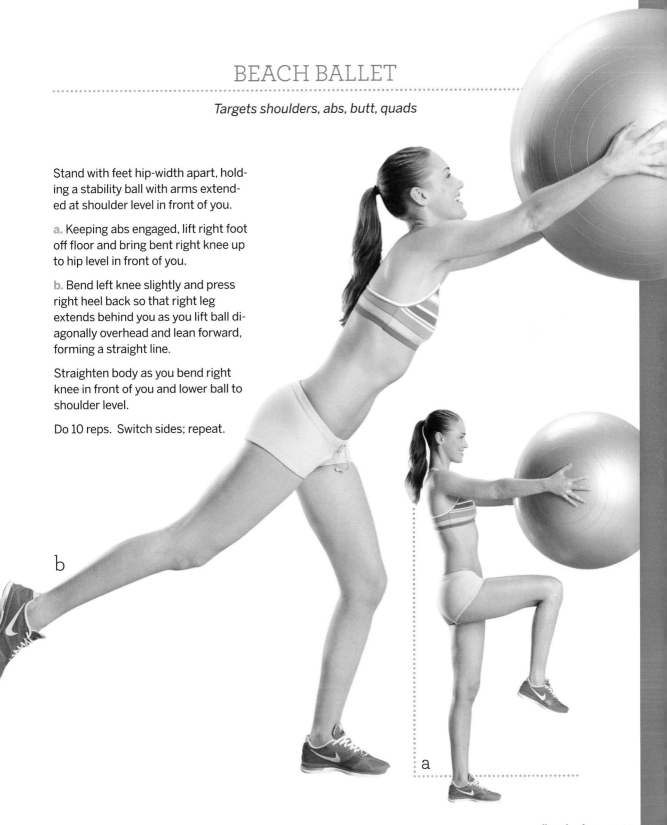

b

a

WRITE YOUR NAME PLANK

Targets abs, obliques

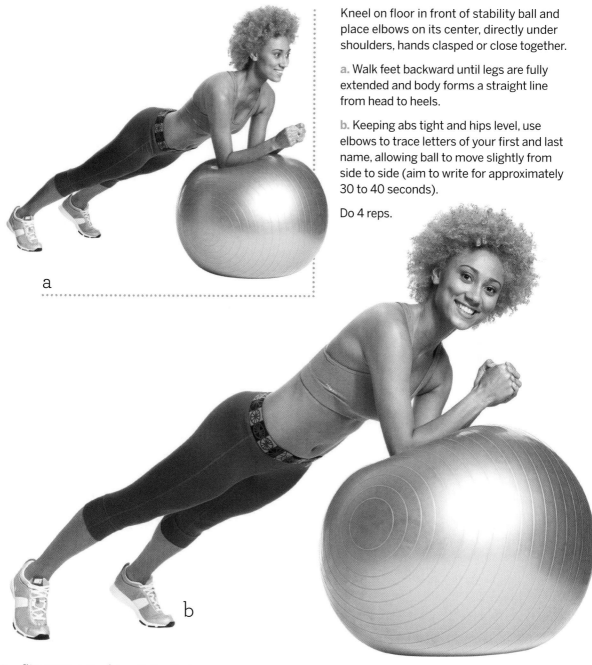

Kneel on floor in front of stability ball and place elbows on its center, directly under shoulders, hands clasped or close together.

a. Walk feet backward until legs are fully extended and body forms a straight line from head to heels.

b. Keeping abs tight and hips level, use elbows to trace letters of your first and last name, allowing ball to move slightly from side to side (aim to write for approximately 30 to 40 seconds).

Do 4 reps.

a

b

BALL CRUNCH

Targets abs, hips, thighs

Sit on stability ball and walk feet out and forward of knees, sliding butt down so body is at a slight incline.

Press palms together in front of chest, keeping a tennis ball–size space under chin.

Pressing lower back into ball, lift upper body and crunch up. Hold for 1 count and return to starting position.

Do 10 to 12 reps.

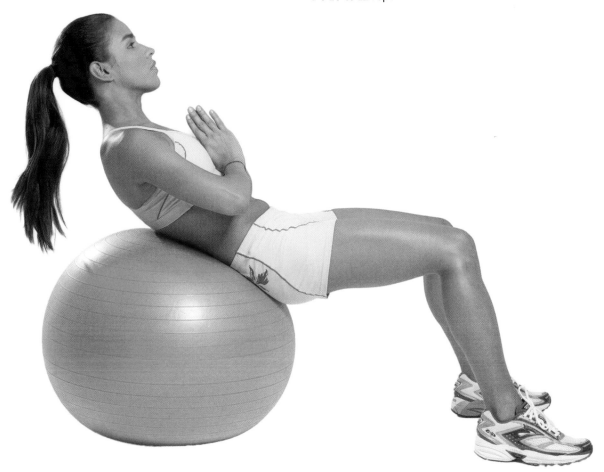

SIDE WALL CRUNCH

Targets abs, obliques

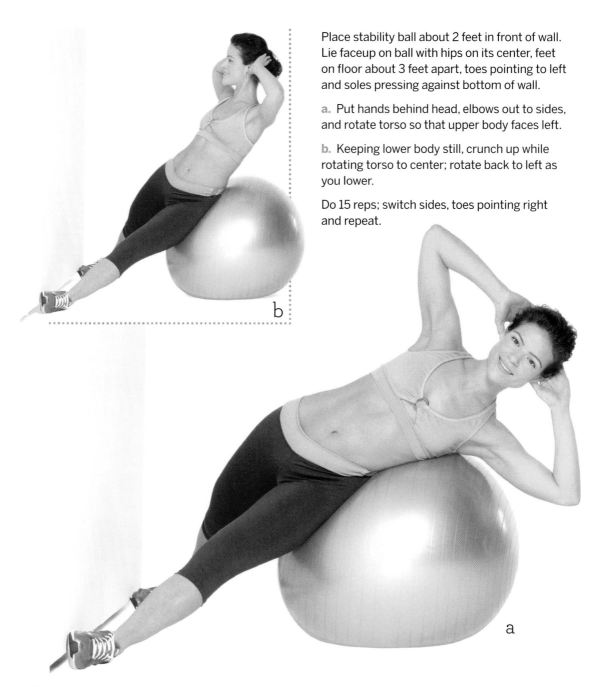

Place stability ball about 2 feet in front of wall. Lie faceup on ball with hips on its center, feet on floor about 3 feet apart, toes pointing to left and soles pressing against bottom of wall.

a. Put hands behind head, elbows out to sides, and rotate torso so that upper body faces left.

b. Keeping lower body still, crunch up while rotating torso to center; rotate back to left as you lower.

Do 15 reps; switch sides, toes pointing right and repeat.

b

a

REVERSE BALL CRUNCH

Targets abs

Lie faceup on floor with legs extended, holding ball between feet, arms by sides. Keeping upper body on mat, bend knees toward chest so that they're directly over hips, calves parallel to floor.

Engage abs and simultaneously lift ball, lower back and hips off floor.

Lower, then roll ball back to start.

Do 15 reps.

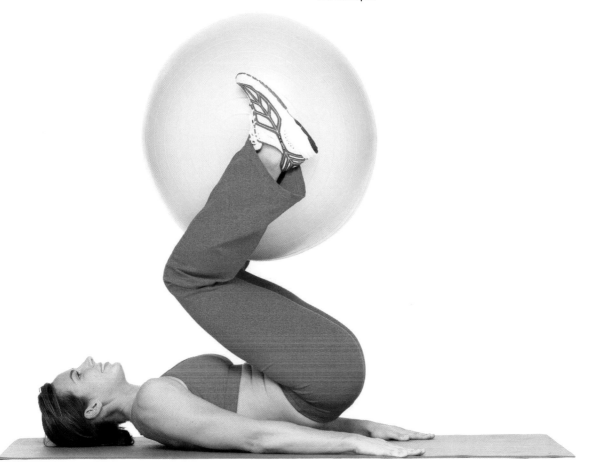

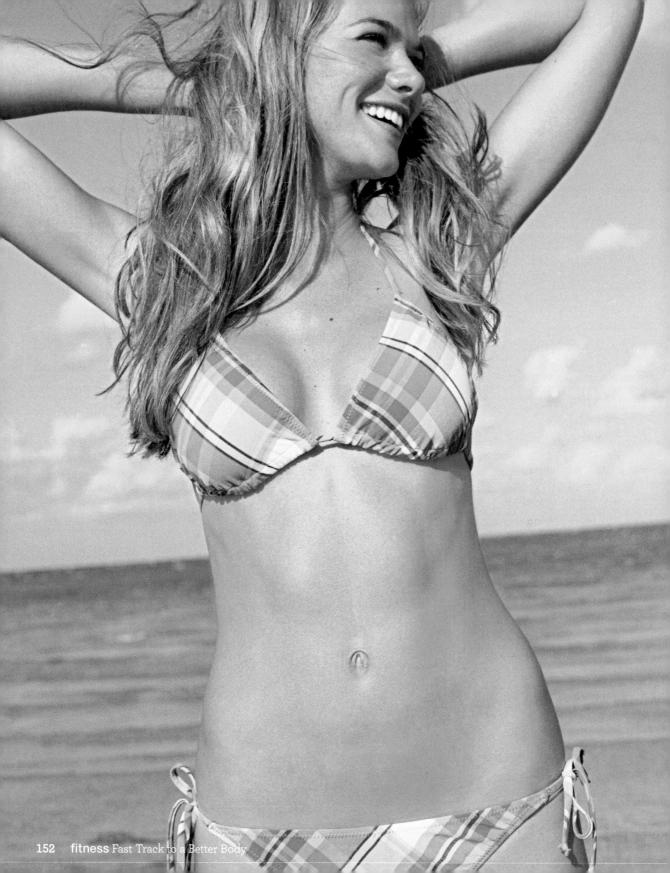

Flat Abs Diet

Light, easy meals that help shrink your waistline

When it comes to erasing flab from around your waist, low-calorie noshes are not created equal. Certain foods contain properties that help zap fat faster. (Think of it as multitasking as you munch.)

These nutrition secret weapons are what help make up the menus in the Flat Abs Diet on the next six pages:

Eggs and Fish: The high protein content of these foods curbs hunger and boosts your calorie burn, so you'll eat less and lose weight.

Milk: The calcium in dairy products trims your waist by increasing the activity of enzymes that break down fat cells. It also reduces levels of the stress hormone cortisol, which causes your body to hang on to belly flab.

Whole Grains and Leafy Greens: Both are loaded with filling fiber, which has been proven to reduce your calorie intake. People on a low-calorie diet that was high in whole grains dropped 8 to 11 pounds and lost more belly fat than those on a traditional low-cal plan, according to a study at Pennsylvania State University.

Mono- and Polyunsaturated Fats: These healthy dietary fats prevent abdominal fat from accumulating in the first place, research shows. You'll find them worked into the Flat Abs Diet in the form of olive oil, fish and nuts—that includes peanut butter!

Try the quickie recipes on these pages, aiming for a total of 1,500 calories a day: Pick one 300-calorie breakfast, one 400-calorie lunch, one 500-calorie dinner and two 150-calorie snacks. Mix, match and slim down!

Did You Know? ACETIC ACID, THE MAIN COMPONENT OF VINEGAR, STIMULATES FAT OXIDATION IN THE LIVER, HELPING REDUCE BODY FAT, SAY SCIENTISTS. IN A RECENT STUDY, OBESE PEOPLE WHO CONSUMED TWO TABLESPOONS OF VINEGAR DAILY LOST AN AVERAGE OF 5 PERCENT MORE BELLY FLAB THAN THOSE WHO DIDN'T EAT IT.

Breakfasts (about 300 calories each)

Strawberry Cereal with a Hard-Boiled Egg

Top ¾ cup Multi-Bran Chex with ½ cup fresh strawberries that have been cut in half and 4 ounces skim milk. Serve cereal and berries with 1 hard-boiled egg on the side.

Vanilla Yogurt with Fruit and Almonds

Combine 8 ounces light vanilla yogurt with 1 teaspoon honey, a splash of lemon juice and 2 tablespoons slivered almonds. Gently fold in 1 cup mixed cantaloupe and pineapple chunks.

Melon, Muffin and Cottage Cheese

Cut a cantaloupe in half and fill with ¼ cup low-fat (1%) cottage cheese. (Use the other half of the cantaloupe in the Vanilla Yogurt breakfast recipe above.) Serve with 1 small low-fat bran muffin.

Pancakes with Banana

Top 2 whole-wheat pancakes with 1 medium banana, sliced, and 1½ tablespoons light maple syrup. Serve with a 6-ounce glass of skim milk, if desired.

Waffle Bacon-Cheese Melt

Toast 2 whole-grain frozen waffles and top them with 4 slices cooked turkey bacon and ¼ cup shredded light cheddar cheese. Place waffles in a toaster oven and bake 2 to 3 minutes, or just until cheese melts.

Orange Smoothie and Peanut Butter Bread

Pour 4 ounces each skim milk and orange juice into a blender. Add 4 ounces light vanilla yogurt and blend until smooth. Serve smoothie with 1 slice whole-grain bread topped with ½ tablespoon peanut butter.

Scrambled Eggs with Veggies, Cheese and Salsa

Whisk together 1 whole egg, 1 egg white, 1 tablespoon skim milk, 1 tablespoon chopped green pepper and 1 tablespoon salsa. Pour egg mixture into a nonstick pan and scramble. Add ¼ cup shredded light cheddar cheese and cook until cheese has melted. Serve scrambled eggs with a toasted whole-wheat English muffin.

PANCAKES WITH BANANA

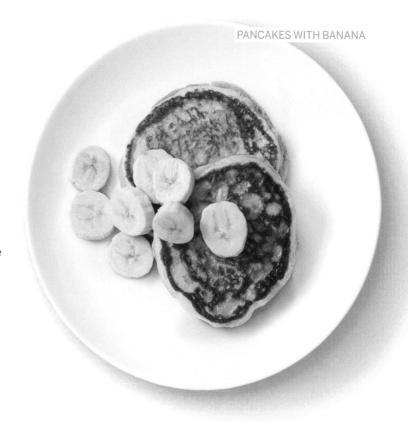

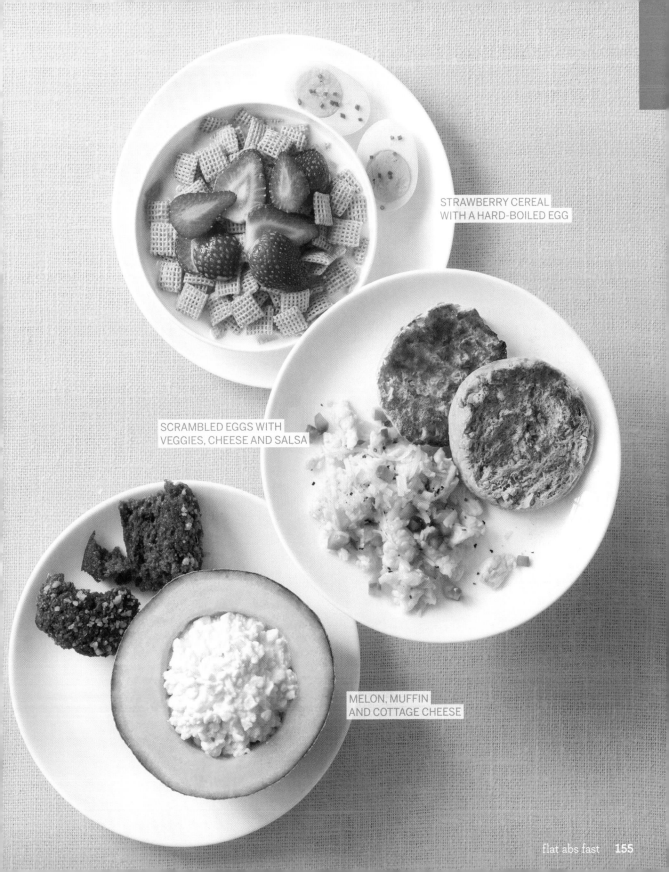

STRAWBERRY CEREAL
WITH A HARD-BOILED EGG

SCRAMBLED EGGS WITH
VEGGIES, CHEESE AND SALSA

MELON, MUFFIN
AND COTTAGE CHEESE

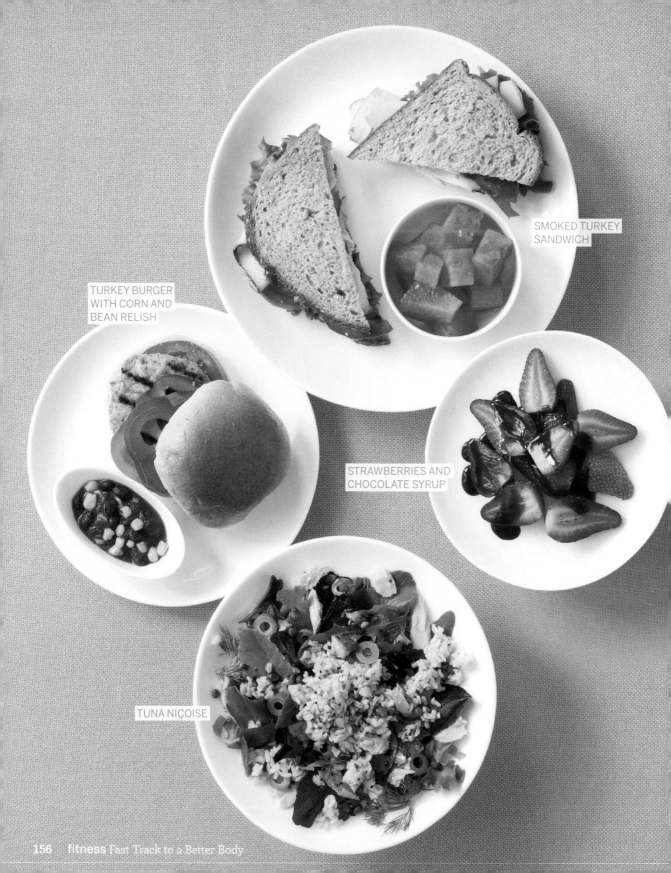

SMOKED TURKEY
SANDWICH

TURKEY BURGER
WITH CORN AND
BEAN RELISH

STRAWBERRIES AND
CHOCOLATE SYRUP

TUNA NIÇOISE

Lunches (about 400 calories each)

Spinach Salad

Toss 3 cups baby spinach with ½ mango, peeled and sliced; 2 tablespoons spicy cashews; 1 cup cooked baby shrimp; and 2 tablespoons light vinaigrette mixed with 2 teaspoons lemon juice. Serve with 1 small whole-grain roll.

Tomato, Basil and Mozzarella Sandwich

Place 2 ounces fresh mozzarella, 1 sliced tomato and a few basil leaves on a small toasted ciabatta roll; drizzle with a little balsamic vinegar. Serve with a medium apple on the side.

Zucchini and Mozzarella Flatbread

Mist a pan with nonstick spray; sauté ½ cup sliced zucchini 3 to 4 minutes. Toast a whole-grain flatbread; top with 1 ounce shredded mozzarella, zucchini, ½ cup diced tomato and 2 tablespoons pesto. Season to taste with red pepper flakes. Broil on low until cheese is melted.

Tuna Niçoise

Mix a 3-ounce can or packet water-packed tuna with 1 teaspoon capers, 6 sliced green olives and 2 tablespoons light vinaigrette; place on 3 cups mixed greens. Top with ½ cup cooked brown rice, cooled.

Smoked Turkey Sandwich

Spread 2 slices whole-wheat bread with 1 tablespoon mustard. Top with 2 slices smoked turkey breast; 1 small tomato, sliced; and lettuce. Serve with 1 cup watermelon chunks on the side.

Tabouli, Beans and Feta

Combine ½ cup prepared tabouli with ½ cup canned white beans, rinsed and drained; 2 tablespoons crumbled feta cheese; 1 tomato, chopped; and ½ small cucumber, chopped. Top with 1 tablespoon chopped fresh mint, if desired.

Turkey Burger with Corn and Bean Relish

Prepare a 4-ounce frozen turkey burger made with 95 percent lean ground meat according to package directions. Place on a whole-wheat bun and top with red and green bell-pepper slices. Combine 2 tablespoons salsa; 3 tablespoons canned corn, drained; and ¼ cup canned black beans, rinsed and drained. Serve with burger.

Snacks

Eat two of these tasty treats a day (about 150 calories each):

- 1 cup strawberries drizzled with 2 tablespoons chocolate syrup
- Celery spread with 1½ tablespoons peanut butter
- 1 strawberry Special K bar and a small apple
- 1 chocolate rice cake spread with 1 tablespoon Nutella
- 1 cup Luigi's Real Lemon / Strawberry Italian Ice
- 1 Skinny Cow ice cream cone
- 1 Minute Maid Soft Frozen Lemonade treat
- 6-ounce Yoplait Light fruit yogurt with ½ cup blueberries
- ½ tablespoon chunky peanut butter on ½ cinnamon-raisin English muffin
- 1 cup carrots, celery and radishes with a dip made from 6 ounces plain, non-fat yogurt mixed with 1 tablespoon onion soup mix
- 1 piece light string cheese and a plum
- Fruit drink: In a blender mix 1 cup frozen peaches and raspberries, 2 tablespoons low-fat whipped topping and 8 ounces zero-calorie fruit punch

Dinners (about 500 calories each)

Tilapia with Pineapple Salsa

Cut 1 medium potato into quarters, brush lightly with 1 teaspoon olive oil and sprinkle with Italian seasoning, basil or oregano; bake at 350°F for 30 minutes. Sprinkle an 8-ounce piece of tilapia with 1 tablespoon seasoned bread crumbs and ½ teaspoon blackened seasoning and broil for 10 minutes. Mix ¼ cup tomato salsa with ¼ cup chopped pineapple and spoon over fish. Serve with potato wedges and 1 cup steamed sugar snap peas.

Chicken and Veggie Stir-Fry

Marinate 4 ounces skinless chicken-breast strips in teriyaki sauce. Stir-fry chicken; remove from pan. Sauté ½ teaspoon grated ginger and ½ teaspoon chopped garlic, add 3 cups frozen Oriental vegetables, and heat through. Add chicken to warm. Serve over ½ cup brown rice.

Steak and Roasted Vegetables

Marinate 4 ounces flank steak in light vinaigrette. Heat oven to 450°F. Place 1 cup sliced potatoes, 1 cup sliced zucchini, ¼ cup chopped onion and ¾ cup sliced mushrooms on a baking sheet; drizzle with olive oil and sprinkle with salt and pepper. Roast 15 minutes. Grill steak.

Asparagus Frittata

Sauté 1 small onion, chopped; ½ cup chopped mushrooms; and 1 cup asparagus pieces until tender. Whisk together 3 eggs, 1 tablespoon water, salt, pepper and a dash of Italian seasoning; pour into pan and cook until egg mixture is set. Serve with 1 small baked potato.

Peanut Noodles with Chicken

Mix 1 cup cooked whole-wheat noodles with 1 tablespoon chopped scallions; 4 ounces cooked, chopped chicken breast, skin removed; 1 tablespoon chunky peanut butter; and 1 tablespoon soy sauce. Serve with 1 cup snow peas.

Shrimp and Vegetable Risotto

Sauté 1 tablespoon chopped onion until translucent. Stir in ¼ cup arborio rice and 1 cup vegetable broth and stir until broth is absorbed. Add 1 cup baby shrimp, 2 cups mixed frozen vegetables and 1 tablespoon grated Parmesan cheese and stir until warm. Mix 1 cup grape tomatoes and ½ small cucumber, sliced, with 1 tablespoon light vinaigrette and serve with risotto.

Rosemary Grilled Chicken

Brush 2 chicken thighs, skin removed, with olive oil; add a squeeze of lemon and 2 rosemary sprigs. Wrap in foil; grill 30 minutes. Toss 1 cup sliced zucchini, 1 sliced red pepper, ¼ cup onion wedges and 1 cup chopped broccoli with 2 tablespoons light vinaigrette; wrap in foil and grill 10 minutes. Serve with ½ cup cooked pasta and ¼ cup tomato sauce.

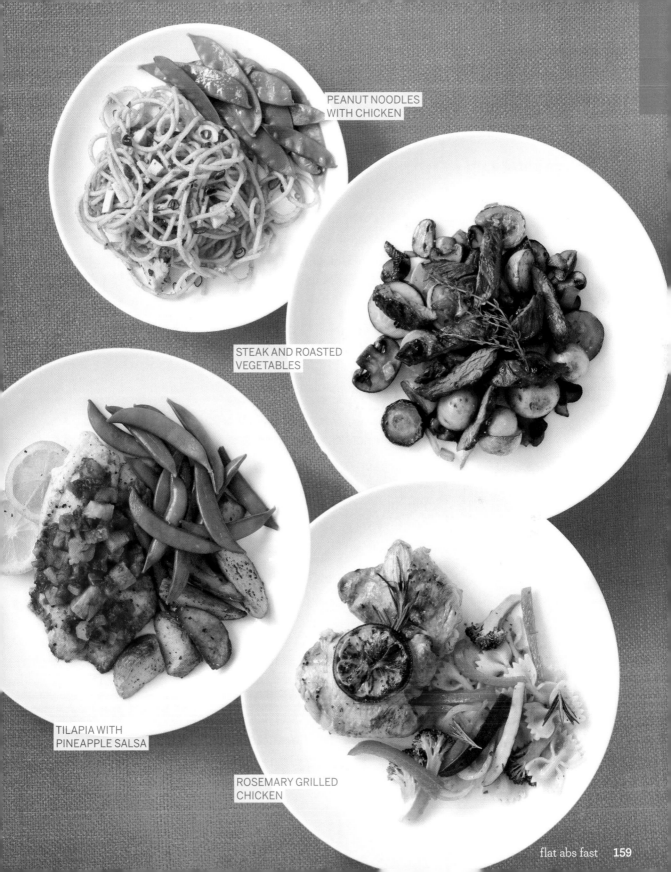

PEANUT NOODLES
WITH CHICKEN

STEAK AND ROASTED
VEGETABLES

TILAPIA WITH
PINEAPPLE SALSA

ROSEMARY GRILLED
CHICKEN

Get a Little Middle

You can practically think your way to a flatter belly.

Sleep it off. Get at least seven hours—preferably eight!—of shut-eye a night. One study found that women who slept only five hours nightly were almost twice as likely to be obese as women who slept seven hours. Research shows that lack of sleep can make you hungrier—it knocks the appetite-regulating hormones leptin and ghrelin out of whack, so you crave sweet and salty snacks. And it can increase levels of the stress hormone cortisol, which causes your body to store fat in your abdomen.

Banish the bloat. FITNESS advisory board member Dawn Jackson Blatner, R.D., gives her four steps to a flatter belly:
Chew slowly—about 20 times per mouthful—to reduce air intake.
Avoid eating salty foods; they make you retain water.
Skip bubbly drinks; they're instant-bloat beverages.
Ditch chewing gum; the action causes your belly to swell with air.

Love your body. Research shows that when women feel bad about their weight and themselves, they're more likely to give up on their diet goals and eat too much. So do things that make you feel good—and that are good for you. Take a walk. Treat yourself to a massage. Go for a bike ride. Before you know it, that extra ab flab will be nothing but a fleeting memory.

Drink in moderation. If you have no more than one cocktail a day, the calories from alcohol will likely burn off. But when you overdo it, they end up turning into ab fat. This is because alcohol inhibits fat-burning in the stomach. As a result, calories from alcohol are more likely to become part of your visceral fat layer, making the possibility of getting a beer (or margarita or wine) gut all too real.

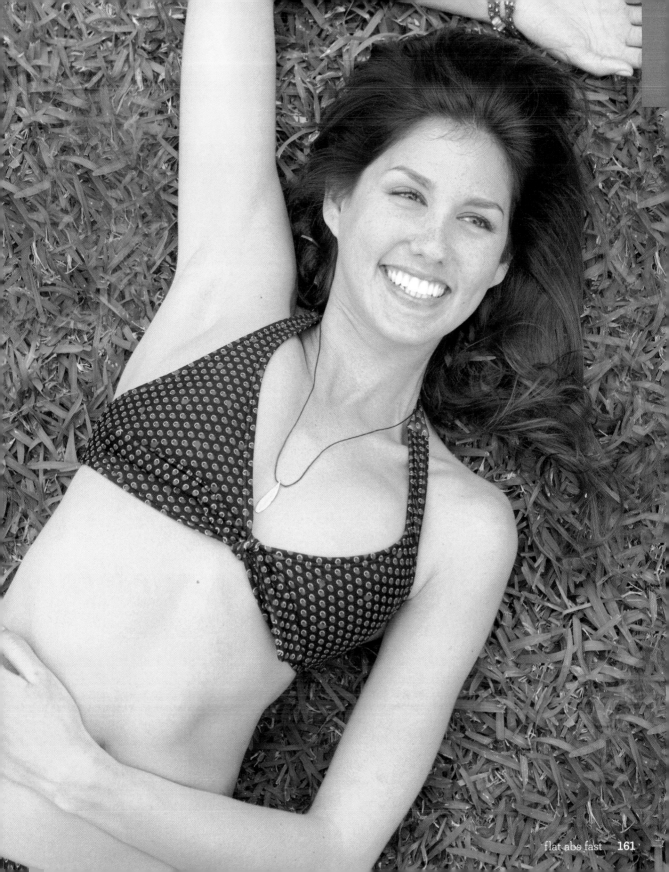

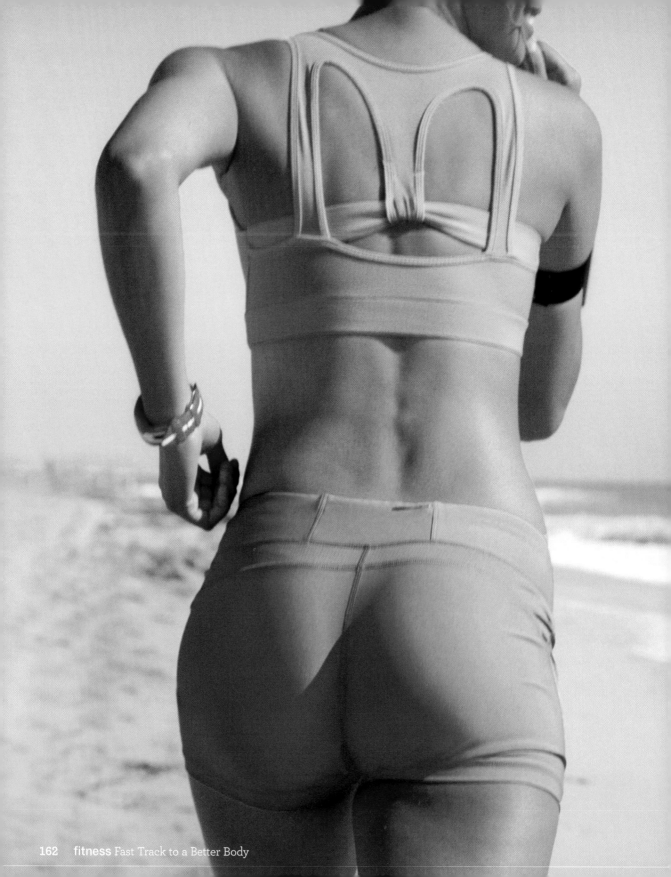

CHAPTER 7

best
butt
toners

LOOK BETTER FROM BEHIND IN NO TIME WITH EXERCISES FOR GETTING A GRAVITY-DEFYING DERRIERE.

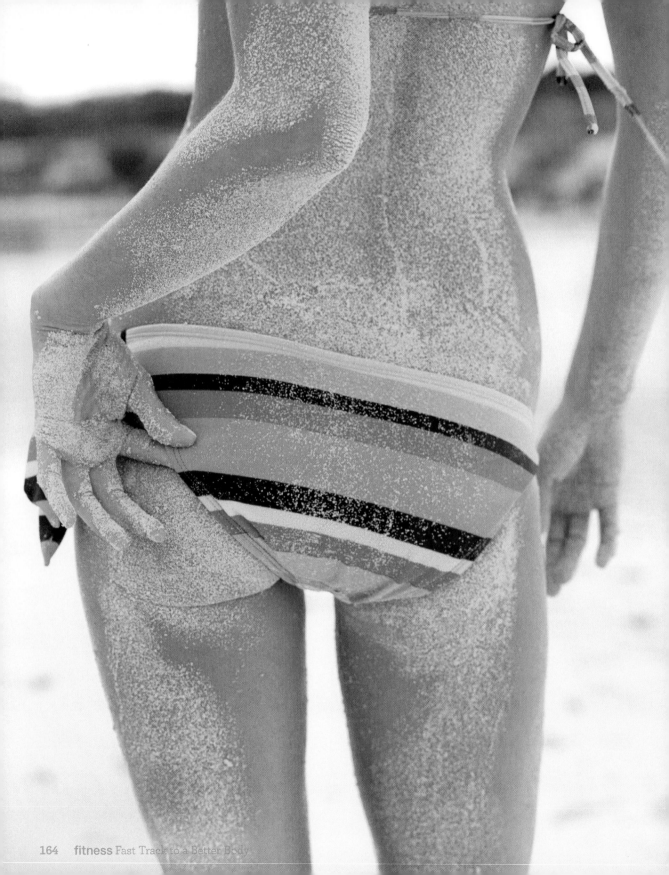

Derriere, rear end, backside, booty, tush—whatever you call your butt, odds are, you've got a love-hate thing going with it. In jeans, you like your rear view. In spandex, not so much. Yet firming your bottom can give your whole body an instant lift. How? The gluteus maximus, one of three muscles that form the butt, happens to be the biggest muscle in your body. Unused, it can cause your whole backside to sag, creating unflattering silhouettes and lumpy panty lines. By sculpting this major powerhouse, you'll stand taller and look slimmer, even if you haven't dropped any pounds.

Step one: Give up your seat—often. "Most of us sit at a desk all day long and totally neglect the muscles underneath us," says FITNESS advisory board member John Porcari, Ph.D., professor of exercise and sports science at the University of Wisconsin-LaCrosse. Too much time spent glued to a chair slows your metabolism and deactivates the gluteus muscles (the medius and minimus round out the trio). The less work they do all day, the harder it is to turn them into buns of steel in your 15-minute workout session. More importantly, the weaker they become, the less efficiently they perform their daily tasks of helping you sit, stand, walk and run.

Because your glutes are such a large group of muscles, sitting on them all day also means your body is burning significantly fewer calories and actually slowing your metabolism. Little adjustments

....

Did You Know?
SIMPLY DOING THREE SETS OF 10 TO 15 ISOMETRIC CONTRACTIONS THROUGHOUT THE DAY WILL HELP YOUR BOTTOM BECOME NOTICEABLY FIRMER: AS YOU SIT, CONTRACT YOUR GLUTES (IMAGINE SQUEEZING YOUR BUTT CHEEKS TOGETHER), HOLD FOR FIVE SECONDS AND RELEASE.

during your day, like standing up from your desk or couch once an hour and walking around, can help keep those metabolic fires going. These may feel like minor moves, but over the course of the day and week, they add up. And it's not only a matter of burning more calories right now, but in the future, too. Since muscle requires more fuel than fat, the stronger your glutes are, the more efficiently your body will burn calories around the clock, even when you're not exercising.

New Rules for Toning

When you think about the moves to firm your butt, chances are, squats are the first thing that come to mind. For years, squats (standing in place and bending your knees 90 degrees to lower into a seated-like position) were considered the gold standard of butt exercises. In a 1999 survey of trainers certified by the American Council on Exercise, the majority of them still cited squats as the best butt blaster.

Since then, new findings have shown that a host of other moves can yield the same, if not better, results, and should be mixed in to your routine. When researchers from the University of Wisconsin-LaCrosse measured the muscle recruitment in exercisers doing a range of butt-strengthening moves, they found that lunges and step-ups engage just as many muscle fibers as the traditional squats. What's more, additional evidence suggests you get the best results from a variety of exercises that can activate and isolate the three gluteus muscles. By working your rear from every angle, as the two routines in this chapter do, you'll see more definition than with squats alone.

Bump Up the Burn

Because your butt muscles lie deep under the skin, the more layers of fat that cover them, the less you'll be able to see the payoff from all those toning moves. Strength training will zero in on this

Q: IS STAIR CLIMBING REALLY THE BEST CARDIO WORKOUT FOR
SHAPING YOUR BUTT?

A: It depends on your technique. "Hanging on for dear life while hunched over the handlebars of a stair climber transfers most of the workload from your glutes to your arms," says Pete McCall, an exercise physiologist for the American Council on Exercise. Touch the rails lightly for balance, or let them go entirely if you can. By not holding on, you'll also burn 30 percent more calories.

muscle group, but the only thing that melts overall flab is cardio. Pick any routine from Chapter 1 to get your cardio dose on most days. If you'd like extra butt-firming from your workout, add an incline. "When you're headed uphill your butt has to work at least 10 percent harder than when walking on a flat surface," says Porcari. "Just make sure you maintain the same stride length when running or walking on an incline as you do when exercising on a flat surface in order to fully extend your glutes and achieve sculpting success." Bonus: You'll burn more calories, too. Using a 5.0 incline during a moderate-paced treadmill walk will blast 346 calories an hour, a 64 percent boost over the same walk without an incline. At a 15 percent incline, you'll burn 60 percent more calories running and 150 percent more calories walking than when you're on level ground.

A second shortcut that will boost the shaping power of your cardio session is to add some speed. Forcing your glutes to contract vigorously, like you do while interval training, will make them stronger than other forms of steady, moderate-intensity exercise, says Porcari. Try out one of the high-intensity interval plans on pages 22–25 or simply add in a few sprints and gentle pickups to your usual walk, jog or bike ride. Start off slowly, then gradually speed up for about 30 seconds until you're almost at a full sprint.

The bottom line? No matter which cardio you choose, do the workouts in this chapter and you're going to love your derriere.

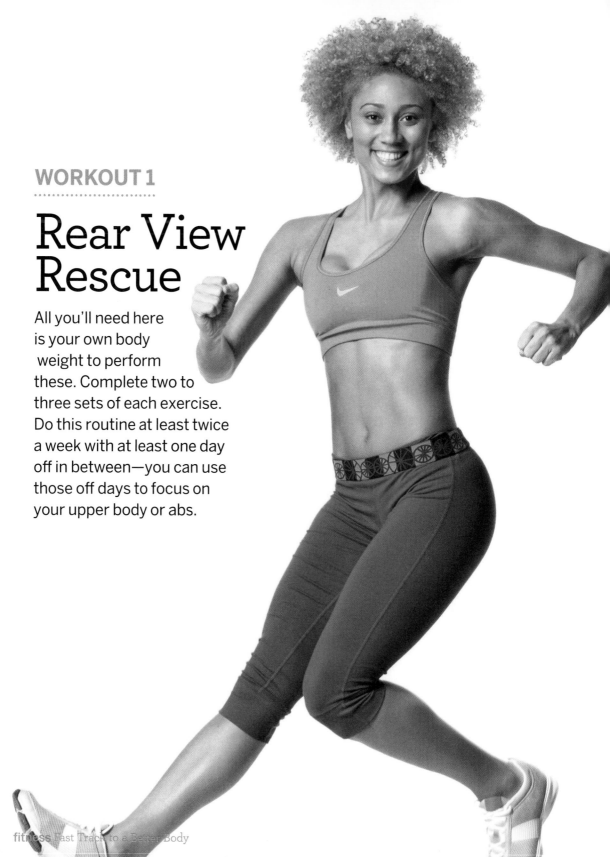

Rear View Rescue

All you'll need here is your own body weight to perform these. Complete two to three sets of each exercise. Do this routine at least twice a week with at least one day off in between—you can use those off days to focus on your upper body or abs.

TREE ARABESQUE

Targets arms, abs, hips, butt, legs

Stand with feet together, arms by sides, abs engaged.

a. Bend right knee out to side, bringing right foot behind left calf. Extend right arm out to side at shoulder level, palm down and left arm overhead.

b. Maintaining arm positions, lean forward slightly from hips as you extend right leg straight behind you, then straighten up as you return right foot to behind left calf.

Do 15 reps; switch sides and repeat.

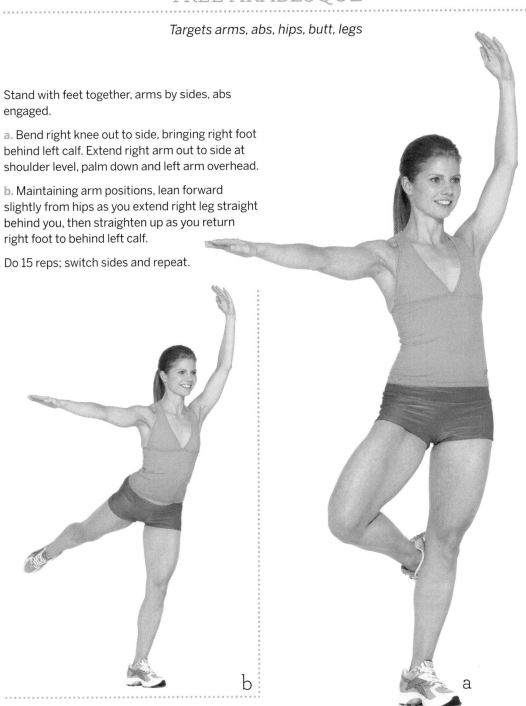

b

a

SQUAT TWIST

Targets abs, obliques, butt, legs

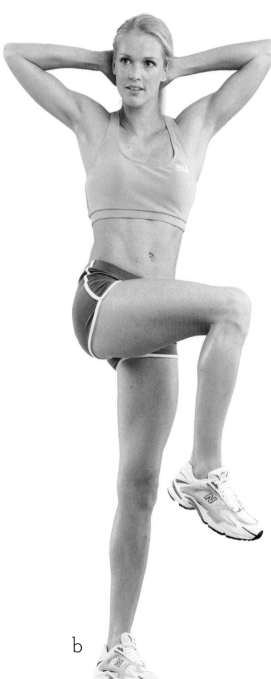

a. Stand with feet shoulder-width apart, abs engaged, hands behind head, elbows out to sides. Squat, keeping knees behind toes.

b. Stand up as you rotate torso to right and lift bent right knee in front of you. Return to squat. Switch sides and repeat to complete 1 rep.

Do 10 reps.

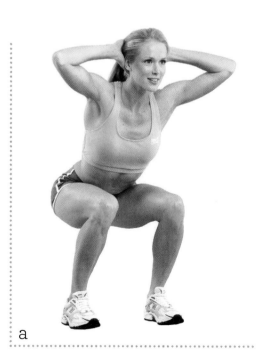

b

a

SLIDE SCULPTER

Targets hips, butt, legs

a. Stand with feet together, knees slightly bent. Hinge forward slightly from hips, put hands above left knee and lift right heel so foot is on tiptoes.

b. Keeping upper body still, extend right leg straight out to side and tap toes to floor, then bring right leg back to start, tapping toes.

Immediately extend right leg straight back, tapping toes to floor behind you; return to start to complete 1 rep.

Do 10 reps; switch legs and repeat.

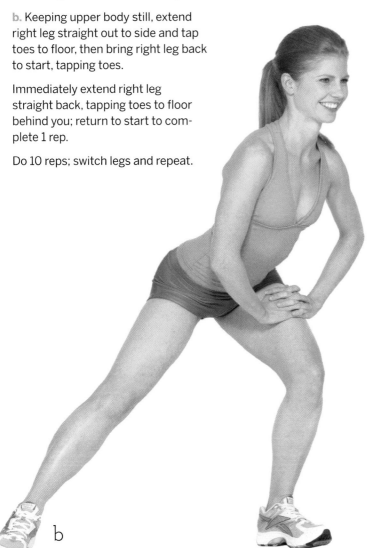

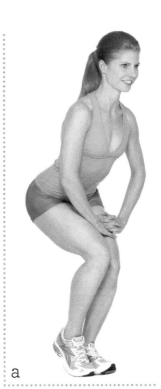

b

a

DONKEY KICK CROSSOVER

Targets butt, legs

a. Start on all fours (hands under shoulders, knees under hips, back flat). Keeping right knee bent, flex right foot and lift knee to hip level behind you.

b. Lower right knee to outside of left knee, then diagonally lift it back to hip level.

Do 15 reps; switch legs and repeat.

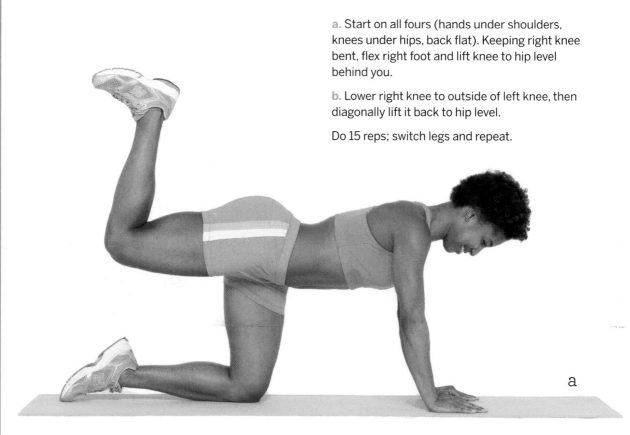

a

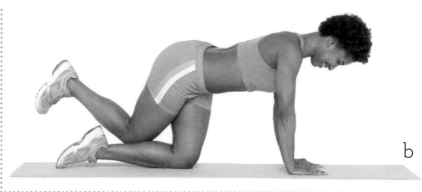

b

GRASSHOPPER

Targets butt, legs

Lie facedown on floor with elbows bent out to sides, forehead on top of hands, and lift extended legs a few inches off floor in a V position, toes pointed out to sides.

Engage abs and press hips into floor. Keeping legs lifted, flex feet and bend knees, bringing legs toward butt. Tap heels together; return legs to V position.

Do 10 reps, without touching legs to floor.

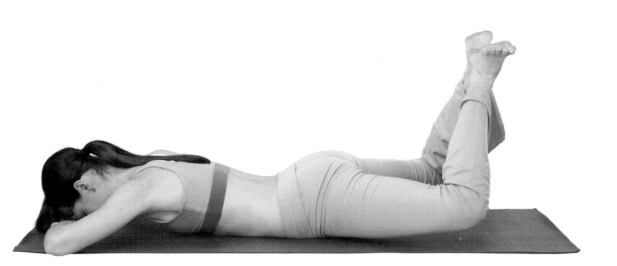

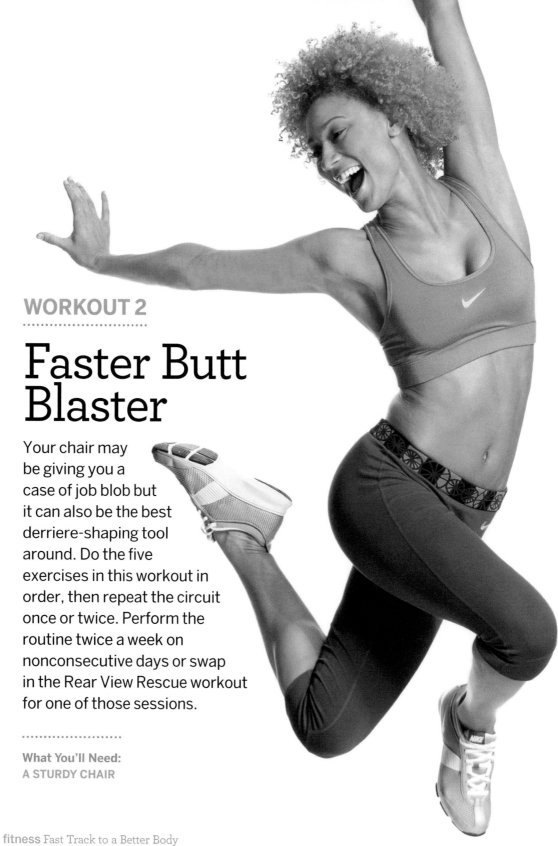

WORKOUT 2

Faster Butt Blaster

Your chair may be giving you a case of job blob but it can also be the best derriere-shaping tool around. Do the five exercises in this workout in order, then repeat the circuit once or twice. Perform the routine twice a week on nonconsecutive days or swap in the Rear View Rescue workout for one of those sessions.

What You'll Need:
A STURDY CHAIR

STEP UP, KICK BACK

Targets hips, butt, quads, hamstrings, calves

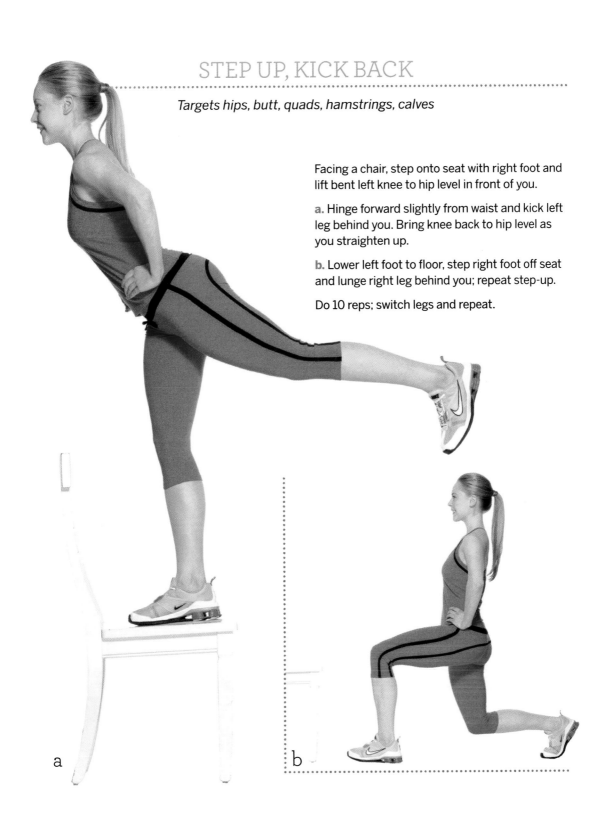

Facing a chair, step onto seat with right foot and lift bent left knee to hip level in front of you.

a. Hinge forward slightly from waist and kick left leg behind you. Bring knee back to hip level as you straighten up.

b. Lower left foot to floor, step right foot off seat and lunge right leg behind you; repeat step-up.

Do 10 reps; switch legs and repeat.

a

b

SEATED SINGLE-LEG SQUAT

Targets hips, butt, quads

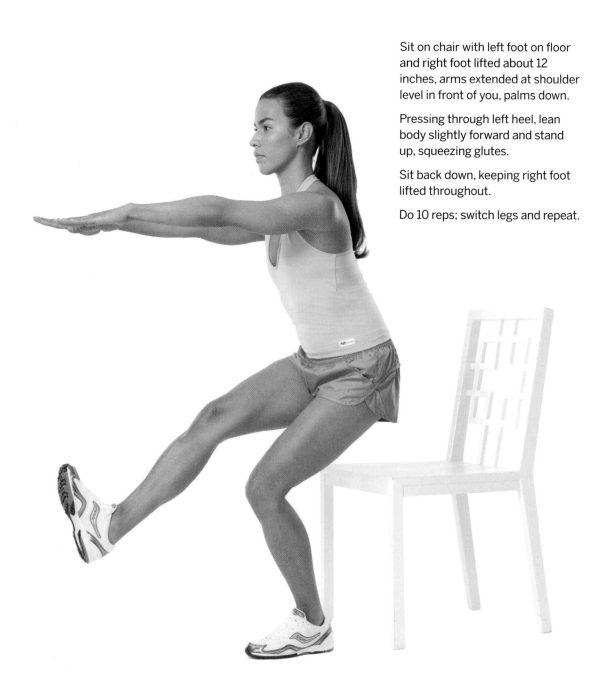

Sit on chair with left foot on floor and right foot lifted about 12 inches, arms extended at shoulder level in front of you, palms down.

Pressing through left heel, lean body slightly forward and stand up, squeezing glutes.

Sit back down, keeping right foot lifted throughout.

Do 10 reps; switch legs and repeat.

ONE-LEG BRIDGE

Targets abs, back, butt, hamstrings

Lie faceup on floor in front of chair with arms by sides, knees bent, heels on chair seat.

Lift right leg toward ceiling, directly over hips.

Keeping upper back and head on floor, engage abs and slowly lift hips until you form a diagonal line from left knee to shoulder. Slowly lower hips to floor.

Do 20 reps; switch legs and repeat.

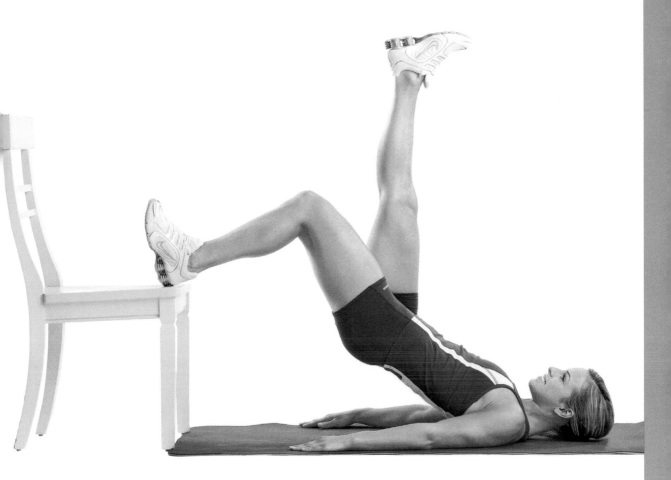

TREE TWIST

Targets hips, butt, calves

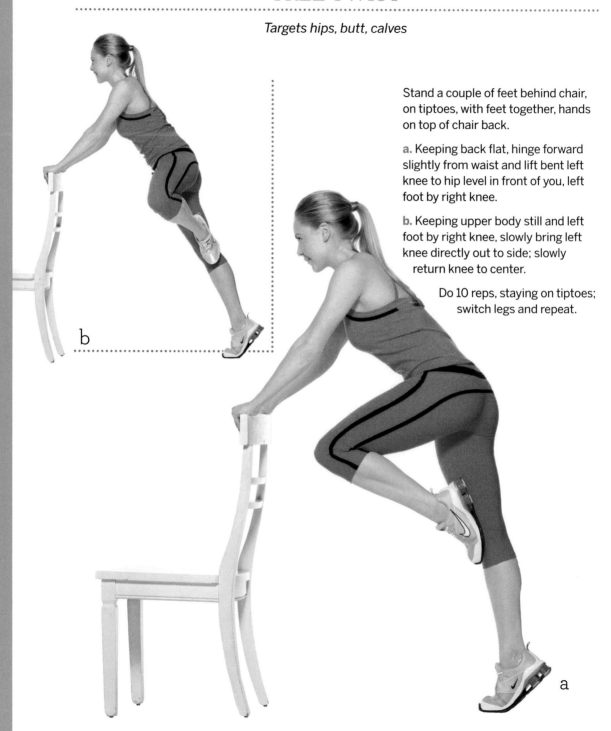

Stand a couple of feet behind chair, on tiptoes, with feet together, hands on top of chair back.

a. Keeping back flat, hinge forward slightly from waist and lift bent left knee to hip level in front of you, left foot by right knee.

b. Keeping upper body still and left foot by right knee, slowly bring left knee directly out to side; slowly return knee to center.

Do 10 reps, staying on tiptoes; switch legs and repeat.

b

a

ROCKING KICK

Targets abs, butt, hamstrings

Stand a couple of feet away from side of chair, with left hand on top of chair back. Extend right leg behind you, toes on floor.

Keeping abs engaged and back flat, lift right leg straight behind you while hinging forward from hips. Touch floor with right hand, then pull upper body up as you lower right leg (like a seesaw).

Do 12 reps; switch legs and repeat.

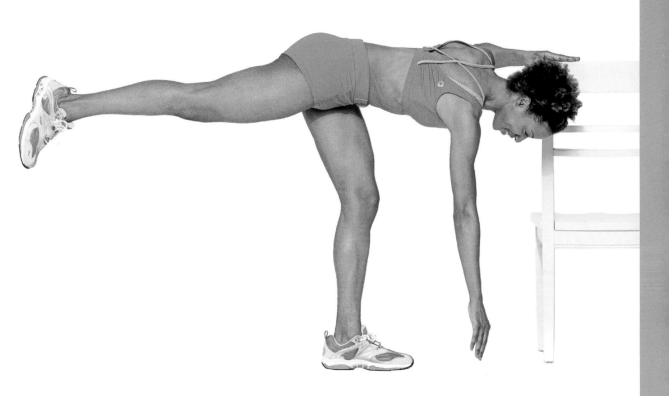

Eat Right for Your Body Type

Got curves you'd like to curb? The trick to lightening your lower half is trimming your fat intake.

It's true that when you shed weight, you do so from all over your body, not just one area. But for classic pear shapes—a larger lower body and smaller upper body—it can be doubly challenging to downsize your derriere. When we drop pounds, our body burns through the fat around our middle first. Which is great, except that pears don't have a lot of belly flab to begin with. Instead, they've got fat around butt, hips and thighs, which refuses to budge.

Some researchers believe this stubborn fat (known as passive fat) is so hard to shed because it was meant to stay put, giving women a ready supply of fuel during childbirth and breastfeeding. Passive fat may actually help reduce your risk of heart disease and diabetes, some scientists say. In fact, fat stored around the hips and butt was recently found to reduce insulin resistance and increase "good" HDL cholesterol.

But if you'd rather lose it than love it, the best way for pears to whittle inches is to watch their fat intake. It's really easy for your body to store the fat that you've eaten, but it takes a lot more energy to store carbs and protein. Because of this, you're more likely to burn those calories off. A diet rich in complex carbs, such as whole-grain cereals, lentils and beans; lean protein, such as chicken or fish; and fruits and veggies will help you to melt off excess pounds.

To see what those foods translate to on a plate, check out the menu on the next page. It's a healthy way to get 1,500 calories a day with the ideal balance of carbs, protein and fat for pear shapes.

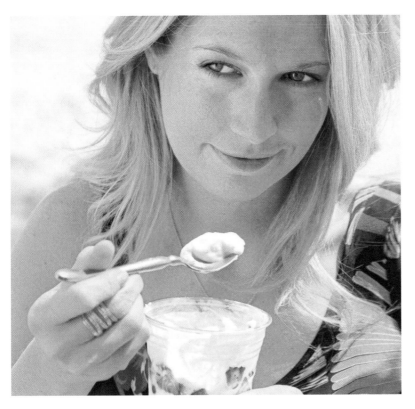

Your Pear-Down Diet

BREAKFAST
- 1 packet instant oatmeal • 1 medium banana • ½ cup orange juice

>

SNACK
- 6 whole-wheat crackers
- 1 mozzarella cheese stick

LUNCH
- Sandwich: 2 slices whole-wheat bread with 1 teaspoon light mayonnaise, 2 ounces lean deli roast beef, 1 slice reduced-fat cheese, lettuce and tomato • 5 baby carrots
- 10 celery sticks • ½ cup grapes

>

SNACK
- 1 cup light yogurt
- 1 small apple

DINNER
- 4 ounces skinless, boneless chicken breast, grilled and topped with a salsa: ½ cup black beans and ¼ cup diced tomatoes • 1 cup steamed green beans • 1 cup mixed green salad and 2 tablespoons shredded low-fat cheese tossed with 1 tablespoon low-fat dressing • 1 whole-wheat roll

>

DESSERT
- 1 sugar-free chocolate pudding cup

Total =1,500 calories: 750 from carbohydrates, 375 from fat, 375 from protein

Mind Over Booty

Love the skin you're in with these feel-good tips from Leslie Sokol, Ph.D., and Marci G. Fox, Ph.D., authors of *Think Confident, Be Confident*.

See the entire landscape. You're more than just a waist, butt and hips. If you let your physical features define you, you risk magnifying them inappropriately. You are a total package, including the emotional qualities your friends love about you.

Poll your popcorn panel. Ask your closest pals what they find most attractive about you. Awkward, perhaps, but a handful of compliments will provide evidence against any self-criticism.

Find middle ground. Like most things in life, how you feel about your body is part of a continuum: Some days you're up; other days you're down. The goal is to minimize the extremes.

Revamp your vocabulary. It's not "I should"; it's "I'm trying to." Relieve yourself of having to live up to a fixed standard you've embedded in your brain.

Use it or lose it. Our bodies are designed to dance, walk, bike and run. Being active automatically brings you joy and enhances confidence, regardless of your shape or size.

Gain Beach Confidence

When it comes to the right bikini bottom, less can be more. "Many women choose a fuller-coverage bottom, thinking it will make their butts look smaller, but the extra fabric can actually emphasize what they're trying to conceal," says swimwear expert Lisa Letarte Cabrinha. Instead, choose a smaller bottom, cut medium-high in the legs and straight across the front, that sits a few inches below your navel.

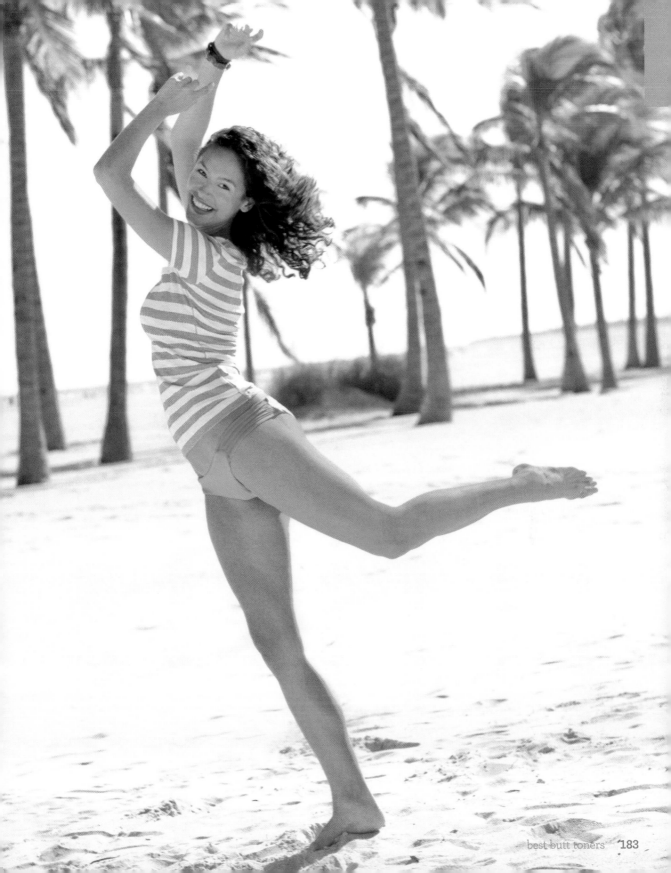

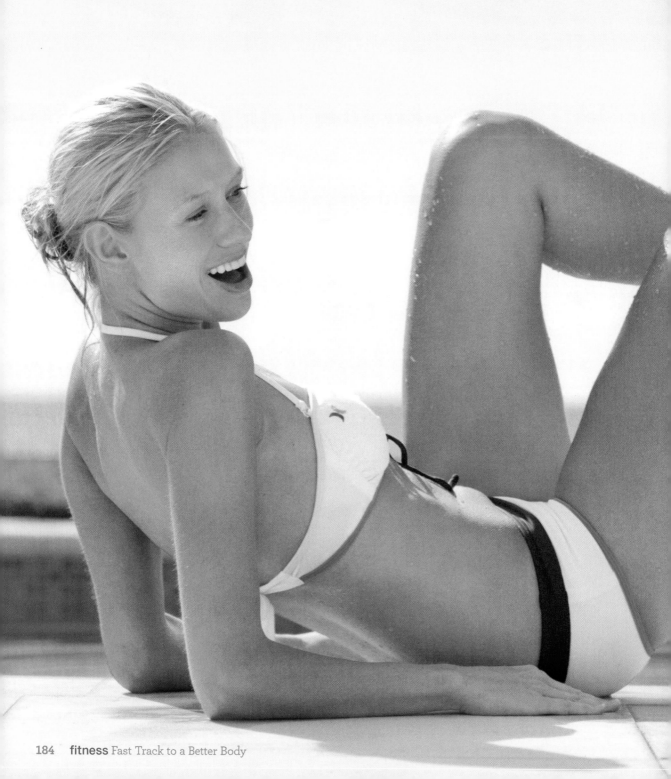

super leg slimmers

FIGHT CELLULITE, FIRM FROM
THIGHS TO CALVES AND
LOVE—FINALLY—YOUR LOWER HALF.

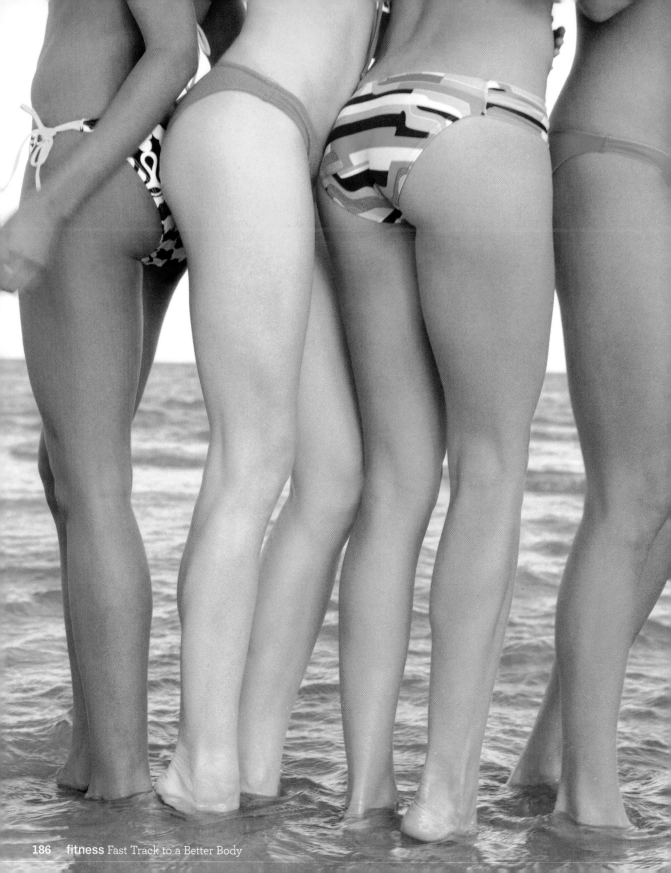

There's nothing like slipping into a pair of short shorts or a mini—or a bikini, for that matter—and loving the way your legs look. But if you're more apt right now to grab a cover-up to disguise your thighs, you're not alone. In fact, fewer than one-third of all women in a recent FITNESS survey said they love their legs, ranking their lower half as a top trouble zone.

Great legs go a long way to making us feel good about our bodies, so why do so many women struggle to tone them? The problem stems from a long-held myth about strength training. "Women worry about bulking up," acknowledges FITNESS advisory board member John Porcari, Ph.D., professor of exercise and sports science at the University of Wisconsin-La Crosse. "Even though it's highly unlikely that you'll develop big, thick leg muscles unless you're doing lots of squats or leg extensions with heavy weights, women hold onto that misconception and avoid working on their legs."

The truth is, our hormonal makeup is not conducive to building Schwarzenegger muscles the way men do. Simply put, we lack the testosterone. In reality, because muscle takes up less volume than fat, developing your legs properly through strength training and burning off extra calories will make them trimmer.

Old habits die hard, however, and many women still dodge the workouts and think they can diet their way to sexy legs. Nope.

Did You Know? IN AVID RUNNERS, THE OUTER QUAD MUSCLE IS OFTEN MORE DEVELOPED THAN THE INNER AND LOWER QUADS, CAUSING STRAIN ALONG THE OUTSIDE OF THE KNEES, SAYS MARTY JAMARILLO, FOUNDER OF I.C.E. SPORTS THERAPY IN NEW YORK CITY. TO STRENGTHEN THOSE WEAKER MUSCLES, DO SQUATS WHILE SQUEEZING A BALL BETWEEN YOUR THIGHS.

Dieting will slim you all over, but it won't get you the contoured Hollywood gams you're after. Only exercise—the right moves in the right combination—will sculpt those, and here's the 3-step recipe:

Step one: Strength-train. Aim to do about two days a week of leg-firming exercises—as with any toning routine, you want to take at least one day off between sessions to allow your leg muscles time to recover and repair themselves before you tax them again. You won't need any fancy gym equipment: Exercises that use just your body weight, like lunges, work just as well as weight machines to give your legs the definition you want, says Porcari.

Step two: Stretch it out. Research shows that beginners can boost strength gains by up to 22 percent when they stretch after weight training. Limbering up could make the difference between staying healthy and sitting on the sidelines. "Tight hamstrings can cause scar tissue to develop, which makes you more prone to injuries," says FITNESS advisory board member Vonda Wright, M.D., an orthopedic surgeon at the University of Pittsburgh Medical Center. (Check out Chapter 3 for a great stretch for hamstrings—and all your other body parts.)

Step three: Get your heart going. To lose jiggle on your legs, you can't forget to do your cardio exercise. It won't target specific muscles the way strength training does, but it will help you burn fat in general. (See Chapter 1 for the scoop on how much cardio to do every week.) One of the easiest ways to score extra leg-shaping from your cardio workout is to vary the routine you do every day. Even if you're a bike devotee and hate to skip a day in the saddle, running one day and hopping on the stair climber or the elliptical trainer another forces your body to use other leg muscle fibers and stay on alert, not autopilot. "By constantly changing the type of exercise you do, you'll challenge your muscles to adapt, which burns more calories and gets faster results," Porcari says.

Q: IS IT TRUE THAT CERTAIN EXERCISES LIKE SPINNING WILL BULK UP MY LEGS?

A: Absolutely not, says FITNESS advisory board member Michele Olson, Ph.D., a professor of exercise science at Auburn University at Montgomery in Alabama. Cardio machines build muscular endurance, not size, says Olson. If you look really closely, it might appear that your thighs are slightly larger immediately after a workout on the spin bike. This is because the arteries and veins in your legs dilate during exercise due to increased blood flow. But the effect quickly diminishes as soon as your heart rate and blood pressure fall back to normal. In the long term, says Olson, cycling or spinning three days a week along with other sculpting moves will leave you with firmer, trimmer legs.

So Long, Cellulite

All of this leg work has another happy side effect: Reducing the appearance of cellulite, which plagues nearly 90 percent of women. More than any other beauty concern, cellulite ranked number one in a recent FITNESS poll; in fact, almost 60 percent of women said they've worn a cover-up over their swimsuit to avoid showing their dimply thighs.

Those dimples are caused by fat cells that manage to squeeze between the bands of connective tissue attaching your muscle to your skin. In addition to looking unattractive, cellulite can also interfere with your flab-fighting efforts by creating a net of fibrous tissue that makes it difficult for the blood supply to reach your body's fat stores. If the blood can't get in, the fat can't be broken down and carried out. While there are plenty of lotions and potions out there that promise to get rid of cellulite, experts agree that the most effective strategy is exercising to shed flab and build muscle, which can shrink your fat cells, making your skin smoother and your legs more toned.

Inspired? Use this chapter as your toolkit for getting the wow legs you've been wishing for. Alternate the two targeted workouts here each week or stick with your favorite for fab results.

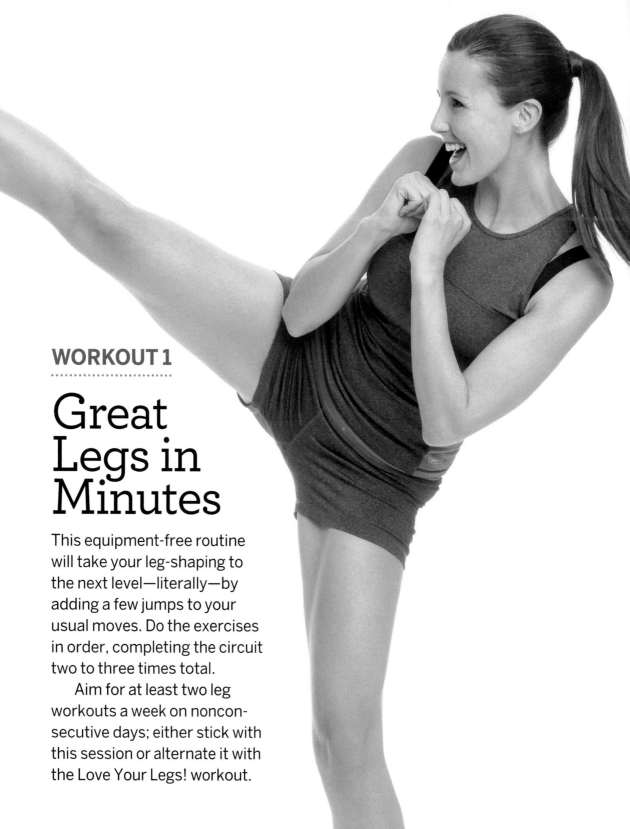

Great Legs in Minutes

This equipment-free routine will take your leg-shaping to the next level—literally—by adding a few jumps to your usual moves. Do the exercises in order, completing the circuit two to three times total.

Aim for at least two leg workouts a week on nonconsecutive days; either stick with this session or alternate it with the Love Your Legs! workout.

SIDE LUNGE JUMP

Targets butt, legs

Stand with feet hip-width apart, knees slightly bent, hands on hips.

a. Lunge right leg to right side, bending right knee 90 degrees and keeping left leg straight, hinging forward slightly from hips.

Step right leg back to start.

b. Do a half-squat, with knees slightly bent, then immediately jump straight up with both feet, bending elbows by sides so fists are in front of chest; land in half-squat.

Switch legs and repeat to complete 1 rep.

Do 10 reps.

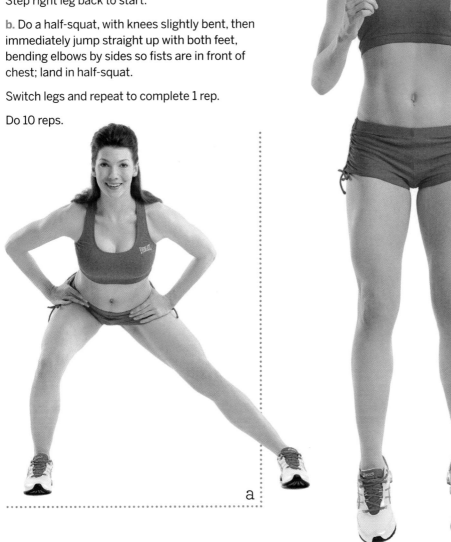

a

b

CALF RAISE SQUAT

Targets butt, thighs, calves

Stand with feet shoulder-width apart, knees slightly bent, arms extended at shoulder level in front of you, palms down.

Squat slowly, keeping knees behind toes and abs engaged, hinging forward slightly from hips.

Hold squat and lift left heel off floor (on tiptoes); lower and lift right heel off floor; lower. Squeeze glutes to stand back up.

Do 10 reps. Switch sides and repeat.

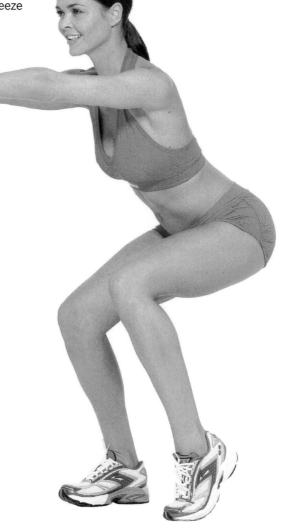

KNEE-UP JUMP LUNGE

Targets abs, butt, legs

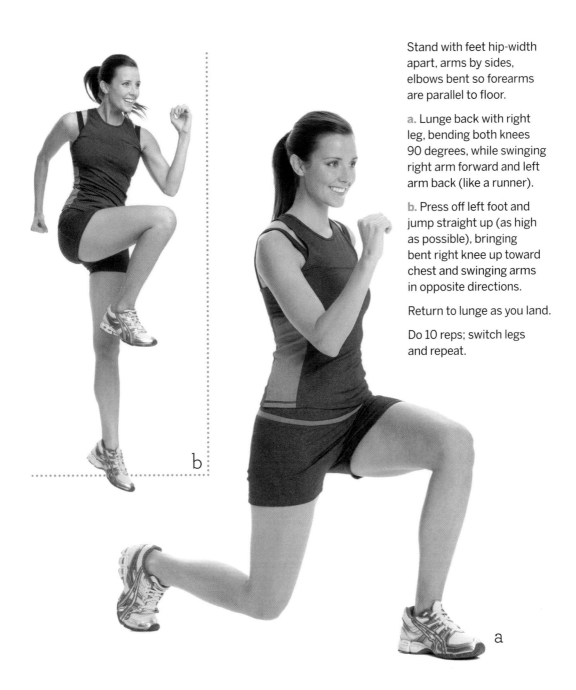

Stand with feet hip-width apart, arms by sides, elbows bent so forearms are parallel to floor.

a. Lunge back with right leg, bending both knees 90 degrees, while swinging right arm forward and left arm back (like a runner).

b. Press off left foot and jump straight up (as high as possible), bringing bent right knee up toward chest and swinging arms in opposite directions.

Return to lunge as you land.

Do 10 reps; switch legs and repeat.

PLIÉ SQUAT JUMP

Targets butt, hamstrings, quads, calves

Stand with feet more than shoulder-width apart, toes pointed out to sides 45 degrees, hands on hips.

a. Lift heels off floor (rise on tiptoes) and squat, keeping knees behind toes, abs engaged and back flat.

Squeeze glutes to stand up; lower heels.

b. Do 15 reps; then do 15 more reps, jumping straight up with legs wide between each squat.

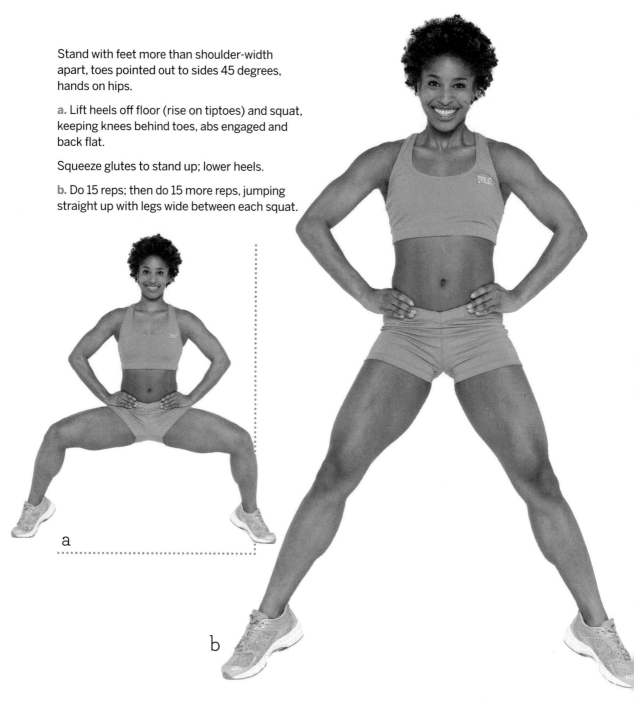

a

b

DIAMOND

Targets abs, butt, inner thighs

Lie faceup on floor with legs together, arms by sides. Lift legs directly over hips with heels together, feet flexed and toes pointed out to sides 45 degrees.

a. Bend knees out to sides (like a frog), bringing soles together.

b. Extend legs out to sides as far as possible, then squeeze inner thighs, pulling legs together over hips.

Do 15 reps, then reverse order (split, frog, start) and do 15 reps.

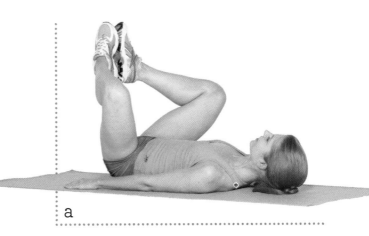

a

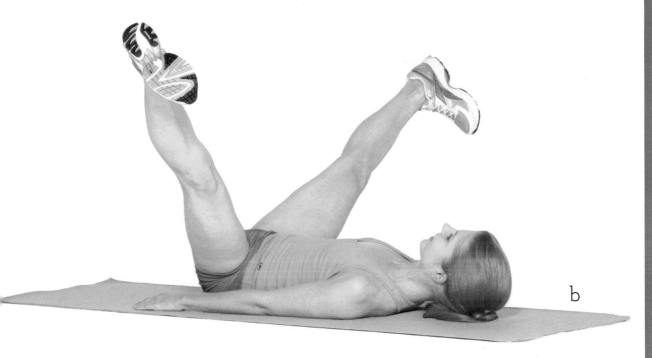

b

Love Your Legs!

Complete the five moves in this workout in order and repeat the circuit once or twice depending on your fitness level. Do this routine two to three times a week, with a day off in between sessions to give your leg muscles time to repair.

What You'll Need:
A STURDY CHAIR

CURTSY LUNGE KICK

Targets butt, hamstrings, quads

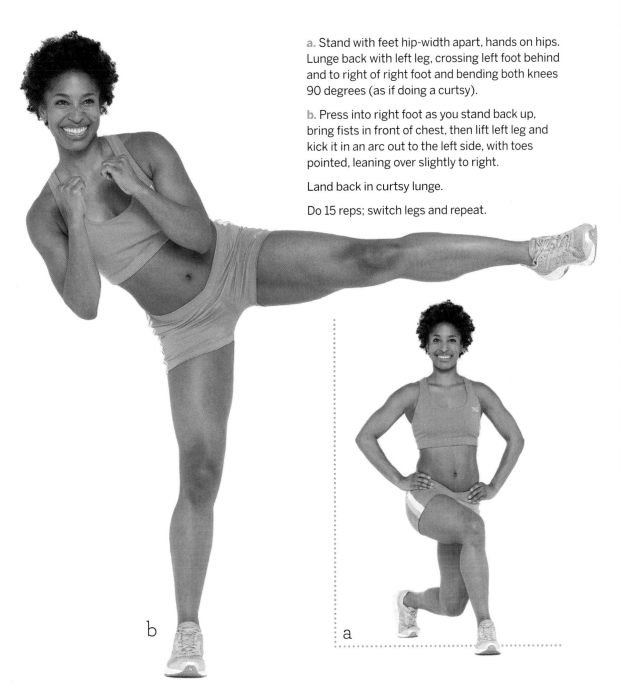

a. Stand with feet hip-width apart, hands on hips. Lunge back with left leg, crossing left foot behind and to right of right foot and bending both knees 90 degrees (as if doing a curtsy).

b. Press into right foot as you stand back up, bring fists in front of chest, then lift left leg and kick it in an arc out to the left side, with toes pointed, leaning over slightly to right.

Land back in curtsy lunge.

Do 15 reps; switch legs and repeat.

b

a

SINGLE-LEG SQUAT TOUCHDOWN

Targets abs, butt, quads, hamstrings

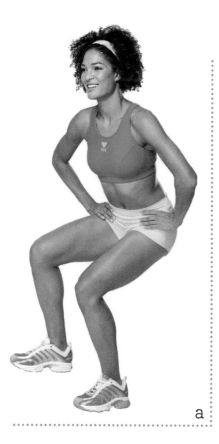

Stand with feet hip-width apart, knees slightly bent, hands on hip.

a. Lift right foot a few inches off floor. Squat, keeping left knee behind toes.

b. Then reach right hand toward left foot with back flat.

Slowly return to start.

Do 15 reps, keeping right foot lifted throughout; switch sides and repeat.

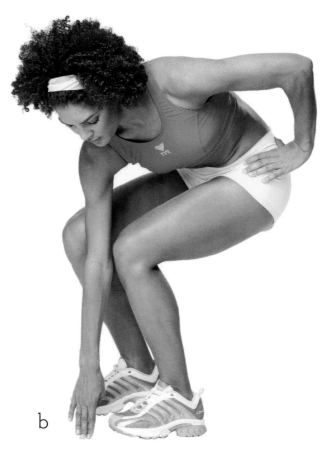

DEMI PLIÉ

Targets butt, calves

Stand with heels together, toes turned out to sides 45 degrees, hands on hips.

a. Bend knees slightly to do a small dip.

b. Immediately rise onto tiptoes, lifting heels off floor.

Hold for 5 seconds, then lower.

Do 15 reps.

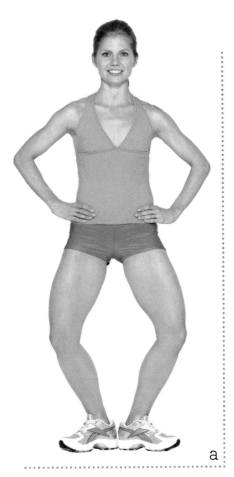

a

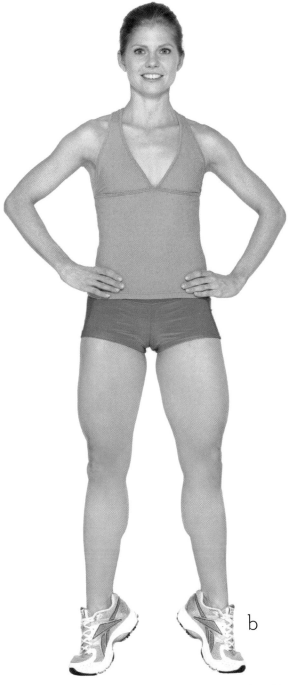

b

ICE SKATER

Targets abs, lower back, hips, butt, outer thighs

Stand behind a chair with feet hip-width apart, gently touching top of chair back for support.

a. Keeping abs engaged, bend left knee slightly and extend right leg out to side, a few inches off floor.

b. Swing right leg behind and as far to left of left leg as possible without touching floor. Hold for one count; extend right leg back out to right side.

Do 12 reps, keeping right leg lifted throughout; switch legs and repeat.

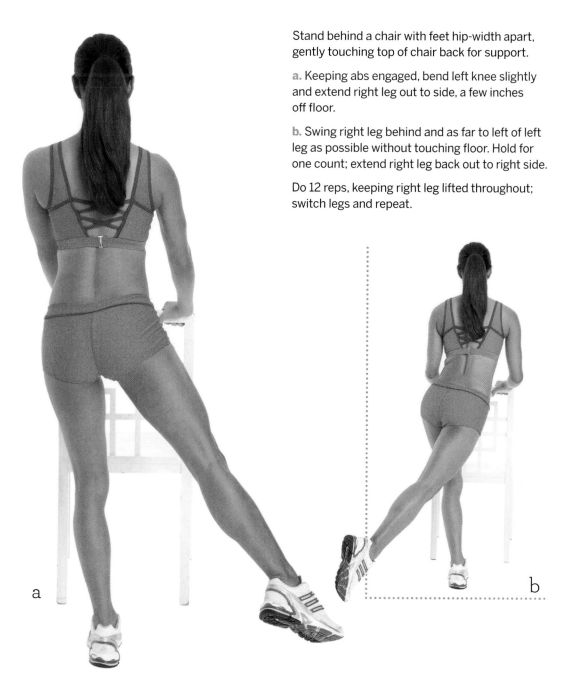

a

b

SQUAT DIP

Targets butt, quads, hamstrings

Stand two feet in front of chair, facing away, with feet hip-width apart, hands on hips.

Lift left leg and place top of left foot on chair seat behind you.

Lower into a single-leg squat, keeping right knee behind right toes and dipping left knee toward floor; straighten right leg to stand.

Do 15 reps; switch legs and repeat.

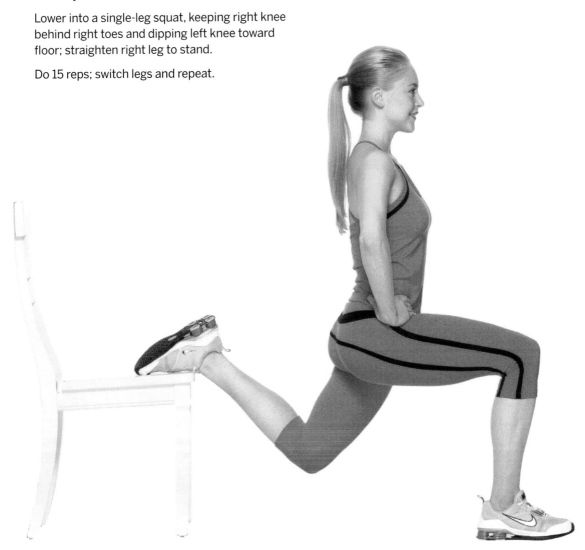

Shortcuts to Sexy Legs

Show off the results of all those lunges by making your legs their smoothest in your next soak or shower.

Scrub your way soft. Give your legs an instant lift by brightening dull skin: Mix ½ cup white sugar (it melts quickly and doesn't sting) with ½ cup olive oil. Then sit in a warm bath for a couple of minutes before you rub a handful of the scrub all over your legs and rinse. "Soaking first breaks up the bonds of dead cells so they fall off more easily," says Cheryl Karcher, M.D., an Avon consulting dermatologist.

Shave to skip nicks. Shave at the end of your shower, when the warm water has expanded pores, bringing hair follicles closer to the surface. "This helps the blade cut hair nearer to your legs," says Shobha Tummala, owner of Shobha Salons in New York City. Use light pressure to avoid irritation and ingrown hairs, and apply shaving cream or oil to help blades glide across skin. It's your choice: With a cream you can see where you still need to shave, while oil shows what you're shaving, says Annet King, a director of training for Dermalogica. If you're using soap, use a cream-based cleanser that contains hydrating petrolatum or a body wash made with sodium lauroyl isethionate, a soap alternative. (When regular bar soap reacts with the calcium in hard water, a gummy coating forms—making skin drier than soap alone, according to Dove research.)

Maximize your moisturizer. To soothe skin and enhance softness post-shave, immediately follow up with a moisturizing body oil or lotion. Warm the lotion in a sink full of hot water while you

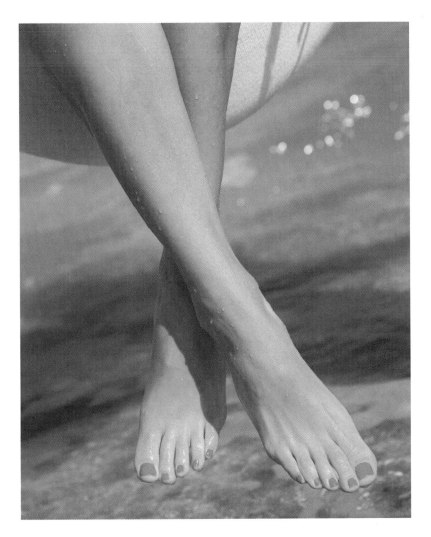

shower or bathe. "You'll be able to massage the lotion in easily, plus the warmth helps it be absorbed more readily," says Donna Perillo, owner of Sweet Lily National Nail Spa & Boutique in New York City.

Protect your skin. Melanomas are more common on the legs in women than men, probably because women want tanned legs and are likely to skimp on—or skip—sunscreen. Rely on self-tanner, not the sun, for color, and top it off with a broad-spectrum sunscreen with an SPF of at least 30.

Eat for Energy

Pump up your staying power while whittling your waist-line with these smart eating strategies.

Before your workout: Pounding the pavement first thing? Have a small snack before you head out the door. Exercising on an empty stomach, especially in the morning when your body has essentially been fasting for hours, can cause dizziness and nausea.

An afternoon gym session doesn't necessarily require a 3 p.m. snack. If you're working out for under an hour, skip it. Or, if you're starving, eat 100 calories of mostly carbs, like a couple of handfuls of whole-grain cereal. If you're going longer than 60 minutes, have a combo of protein and carbs, like toast with peanut butter and banana (200 to 300 calories), about an hour beforehand.

Drink 8 to 12 ounces of water or a low-cal sports drink about an hour before you exercise.

While you sweat: Once you're moving, gulp 6 to 8 ounces of water every 15 minutes or so to stay hydrated. Going longer than an hour? Grab a sports drink, which will give you the electrolytes, fluids and sugar-filled carbs you need to keep at it.

If you're doing a moderately intense workout or exercising for an hour or less, you probably don't need an additional snack. If you are training for an endurance event, you may want to consider energy gels or bars to replenish the energy lost as you continue to run or bike for extended periods of time.

When you finish: Try to eat within 30 minutes post-workout, that's when your muscles are best primed to replace their power supply. An easy way to replenish is with an 8- to 12-ounce glass of chocolate milk or a combo of mostly carbs (75 to 80 percent) with some protein (20

Did You Know? **HIGH-PROTEIN GREEK YOGURT PROVIDES THE AMINO ACIDS YOUR MUSCLES NEED TO REPAIR THEMSELVES AFTER A HARD WORKOUT. BONUS POINTS IF YOU GULP A BOTTLE OF WATER ALONG WITH IT: THE PROTEIN MAY INCREASE THE AMOUNT OF H_2O ABSORBED BY THE INTESTINES, IMPROVING HYDRATION.**

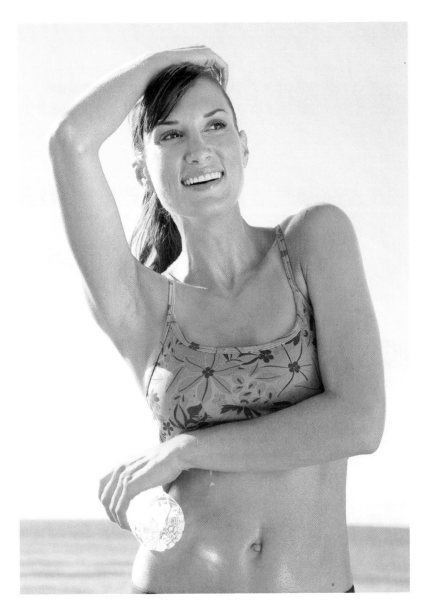

protein (20 to 25 percent), such as a handful of whole-grain crackers with hummus or a few slices of low-fat cheese.

Limit your caloric intake to one-half of what you've burned off. For instance, if you burned approximately 300 calories on the elliptical, have a low-fat yogurt (about 150 calories) or a banana with a smear of peanut butter.

Go Longer and Stronger

During a tough workout or race, when you feel like you've got nothing left, it's tempting to throw in the towel. Don't. Use these three mind games to keep a positive attitude as you move.

Adjust your focus: Yes, running is hard. But instead of zeroing in on how much your quads ache, notice how strong your core feels or how fast your arms are pumping. Called chunking, this distraction strategy shifts your attention to just one area of your body, so the rest of you doesn't feel so tired.

Think small: Counting down the minutes on the elliptical or the number of miles you still have left to bike can make it seem like you'll never finish. Instead, when you want to quit, "tell yourself that you can do anything for two minutes," says Patrick Cohn, Ph.D., a sports psychologist and the founder of Peak Performance Sports, a company that offers mental coaching to professional athletes. "Then gradually increase the time increments to three minutes and five minutes until you're done."

Peel off pressure: A race is an opportunity to showcase how all those early-morning bike rides or Saturday sessions have paid off, but if things aren't going your way, that doesn't mean you should give up. Setting a personal best is not the only measure of success. Remind yourself how hard you've worked to be at the starting line and focus on what you need to do to get to the finish—whether it's taking a quick walk break or grabbing a cup of water at the next aid station.

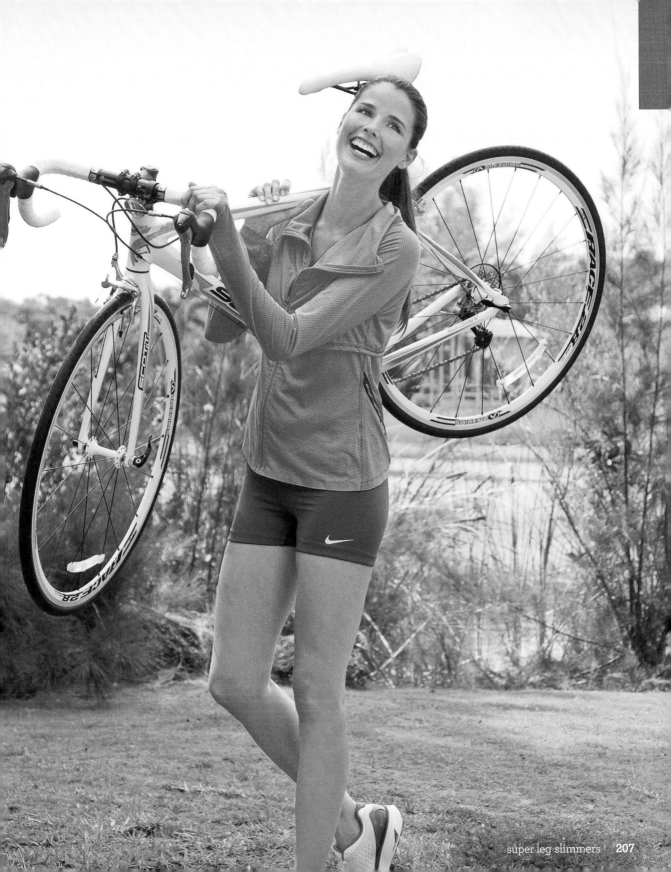

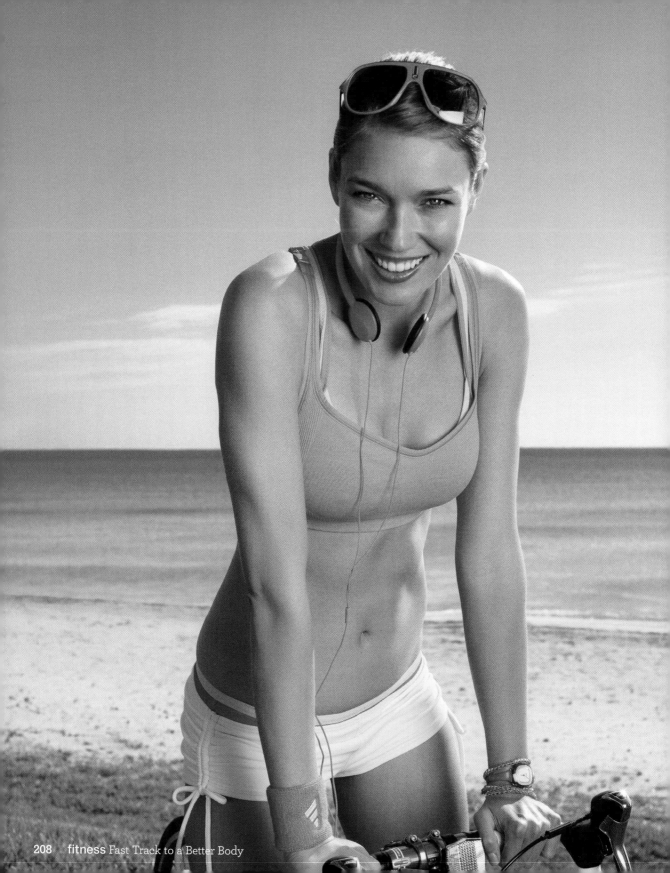

total body workouts

REBOOT YOUR ROUTINE USING THESE
FIVE FRESH COMBOS OF THE
MOVES FROM CHAPTERS 4 THROUGH 8
OR CREATE YOUR OWN MIX.

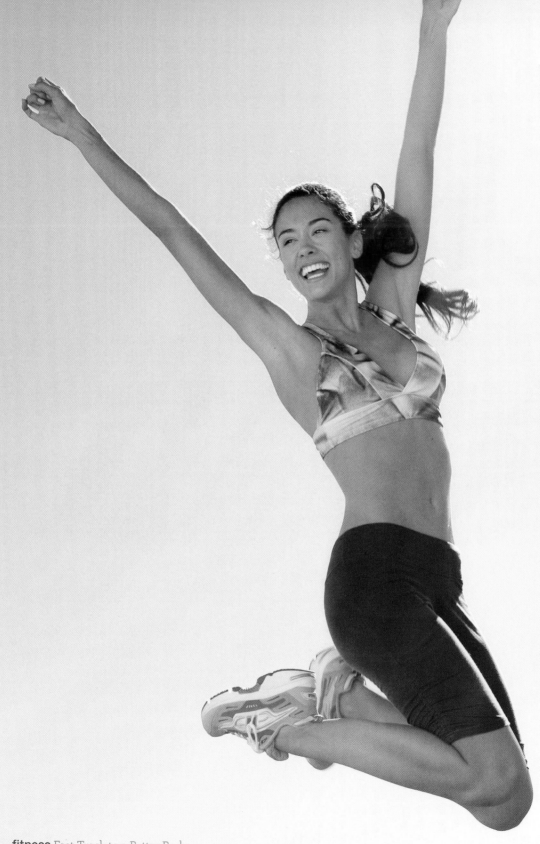

You've just learned 50—count 'em!—new exercises that add up to firm every inch of you from shoulders to shins and abs to calves. In this chapter, we'll show you how to combine and reshuffle those moves to create complete head-to-toe workouts that will take you just 15 minutes.

The best part about these routines: They save you time and stave off boredom, two of the top reasons women cited for falling off the exercise wagon in a recent FITNESS poll. Even the most devoted fitness fan gets sick of the same workout every day. With 50 moves to choose from in this book, the possibilities to change things up are endless. Once you've gone through the routines in this chapter a few times, you can even mix and match your own. Feeling like your legs need a little more attention? Work in some extra moves from Chapter 8. Need to focus on your belly—and biceps? Borrow more from Chapters 6 and 4, respectively.

One more reason you'll love rotating through these routines is that you'll see results faster. Why? Because when you surprise your muscles with moves they aren't expecting, you force them to work harder and therefore get stronger. "It's easy to fall into a comfort zone where you keep doing the same thing even when you're not seeing improvement," says Barbara Bushman, Ph.D., a professor of exercise physiology at Missouri State University in Springfield. "You need to continually challenge your muscles. They

Did You Know?
THAT LAST ROUND OF REPS REALLY PAYS OFF: STUDIES REVEAL THAT YOU'LL SEE UP TO 46 PERCENT GREATER STRENGTH GAINS BY DOING TWO TO THREE SETS (ABOUT 7 TO 10 REPS EACH) OF ANY STRENGTH-TRAIN-ING EXERCISE—UPPER OR LOWER BODY—COMPARED WITH JUST ONE.

will improve only when you ask them to do something they're not accustomed to."

Plus, routines that work multiple muscle groups require the body to operate as it does in real life. "You have to squat down and pick something up while you're holding your purse on your right arm, and balancing in the heel of your left shoe," says Michele Olson, Ph.D., a FITNESS advisory board member and professor of exercise science at Auburn University at Montgomery in Alabama. "It's like doing a squat with a row or a lunge with biceps curls."

In addition to mixing up the moves, you can also vary the number of reps, the amount of rest time you take between sets and the amount of weight you're using. Keep in mind these three basic rules to get the biggest bang from your total body workout.

Rule #1: Be consistent. No matter how you work it (either targeting each body part individually or training all your muscles together), the American College of Sports Medicine and the American Heart Association recommend you do strength-training sessions a minimum of twice a week on top of your cardio workouts to receive the full health (and toning) benefits. Once you get comfortable with two, consider bumping it up a notch. "Doing two strength-training sessions a week is good, but three is even better," says Olson. After age 30, women who do nothing lose about a quarter pound of muscle mass each year. Strength training builds strong muscles, helps boost your metabolism and keep bones healthy. Just make sure you leave at least one day in between each workout to help your body recover. At the end of each week, you'll want to be sure you've hit every major muscle group in at least one of your sessions. That's easy: Simply aim to work in a move (or two) from each chapter.

Rule #2: Go from big to small. To reap the best results out of your total body workout, target larger muscles first. "The larger the muscles you're using, the more blood you've got flowing throughout your body, which helps fuel smaller muscles as you go through your workout," explains Olson. "The goal is to be good and warm by the time you get to those smaller muscles where you'd really like to see definition and tone." For example, pick a move that works your butt muscles first, like the Tree Arabesque in Chapter 7, then progress to legs and abs and finish with a move like the Back Touch in Chapter 5 that focuses on smaller back muscles. Not in the mood to create your own program? No worries! The five total-body routines in this chapter eliminate the guesswork.

Rule #3: Keep it snappy. A long workout does not necessarily make a better workout. In fact, a shorter, speedier session can elevate your heart rate and your fat-burning. "By constantly moving from one move to the next, you're adding a cardio element, revving up your metabolism and burning more calories both during and after your workout," says Olson. This nonstop action, aka circuit training, burns about 25 percent more calories than traditional resistance workouts that have built-in rest periods.

One more thing: Hustling through these short, super-shaper routines will keep you coming back again and again, once you see the time-saving, butt-lifting benefits.

Simple Shape-Up

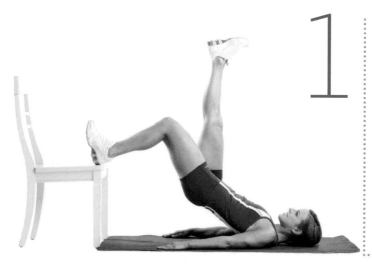

1

ONE-LEG BRIDGE
Targets abs, back, butt, hamstrings

Lie faceup on floor in front of chair with arms by sides, knees bent, heels on chair seat.

Lift right leg toward ceiling, directly over hips.

Keeping upper back and head on floor, engage abs and slowly lift hips until you form a diagonal line from left knee to shoulder. Slowly lower hips to floor.

Do 20 reps; switch legs and repeat.

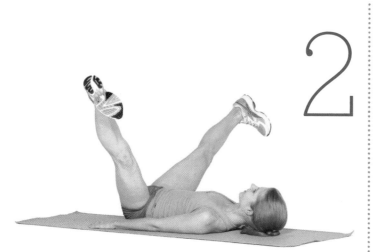

2

DIAMOND
Targets abs, butt, inner thighs

Lie faceup on floor with legs together, arms by sides. Lift legs directly over hips with heels together, feet flexed and toes pointed out to sides 45 degrees.

Bend knees out to sides (like a frog), bringing soles together.

Extend legs out to sides as far as possible, then squeeze inner thighs, pulling legs together over hips.

Do 15 reps, then reverse order (split, frog, start) and do 15 reps.

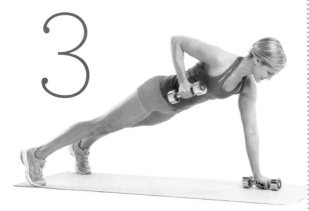

DOUBLE-LIFT PUSH-UP
Targets shoulders, upper back, chest, abs, obliques

Holding a dumbbell in each hand, get into full push-up position (balancing on hands and toes so body is parallel with floor), hands under shoulders, palms in.

Keeping abs engaged, do a push-up, then pull right elbow toward ceiling, bringing dumbbell next to ribs while keeping left arm straight. Hold for 1 count and lower right arm; repeat with left arm to complete 1 rep.

Do 5 reps.

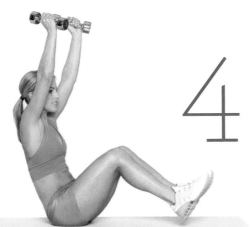

KNEE-UP PRESS
Targets shoulders, abs, butt

Sit on floor with knees bent and feet flat on floor, holding a dumbbell in each hand. Bend elbows by sides, bringing dumbbells in front of shoulders, palms facing in.

Keeping shoulders down, lean back slightly and extend arms overhead as you lift feet a few inches off floor, bringing knees toward chest.

Hold position for 1 to 3 counts; lower dumbbells to shoulders and heels to floor to complete 1 rep.

Do 15 reps.

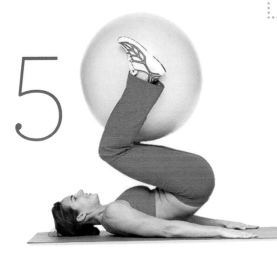

REVERSE BALL CRUNCH
Targets abs

Lie faceup with legs extended, holding ball between feet, arms by sides. Keeping upper body on mat, bend knees toward chest so that they're directly over hips, calves parallel to floor.

Engage abs and simultaneously lift ball, lower back and hips off floor.

Lower, then roll ball back to start.

Do 15 reps.

Flab Fighters

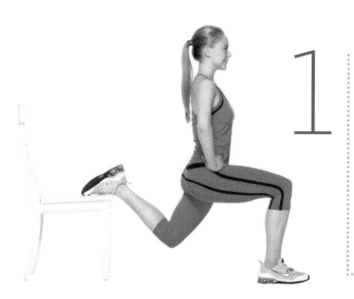

1 SQUAT DIP
Targets butt, quads, hamstrings

Stand two feet in front of chair, facing away, with feet hip-width apart, hands on hips.

Lift left leg and place top of left foot on chair seat behind you.

Lower into a single-leg squat, keeping right knee behind right toes and dipping left knee toward floor; straighten right leg to stand.

Do 15 reps; switch legs and repeat.

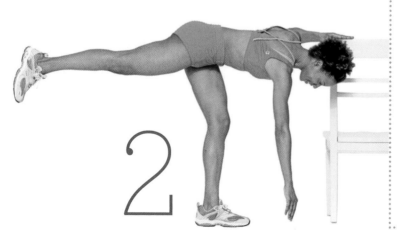

2 ROCKING KICK
Targets abs, butt, hamstrings

Stand a couple of feet away from side of chair, with left hand on top of chair back. Extend right leg behind you, toes on floor.

Keeping abs engaged and back flat, lift right leg straight behind you while hinging forward from hips. Touch floor with right hand, then pull upper body up as you lower right leg (like a seesaw).

Do 12 reps; switch legs and repeat.

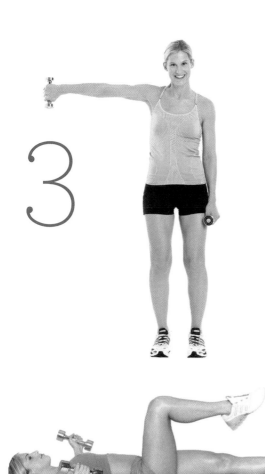

SIDE TRI LIFT

Targets triceps

Stand with feet hip-width apart, holding a dumbbell in each hand, arms by sides.

Bend right elbow by side so that right palm is facing shoulder.

Straighten right arm out to side at shoulder level so palm faces back.

Lift arm up 2 inches; lower. Bend elbow, bringing hand in front of shoulder again.

Keeping upper arm at shoulder level throughout, extend arm to repeat move.

Do 20 reps; switch arms and repeat.

CHEST FLYE BICYCLE

Targets chest, abs

Holding a dumbbell in each hand, lie faceup on floor with knees bent 90 degrees over hips, arms extended directly above chest, palms in.

Keeping right knee bent, straighten left leg toward floor as you lower arms out to sides with elbows slightly bent. Hold for 1 count, then return to start.

Do 10 reps; switch legs and repeat.

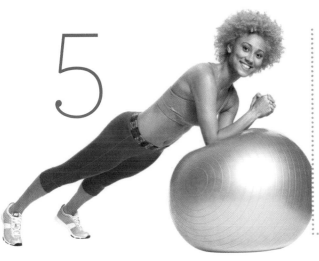

WRITE YOUR NAME PLANK

Targets abs, obliques

Kneel on floor in front of stability ball and place elbows on its center, clasping hands together.

Walk feet backward until legs are fully extended and body forms a straight line from head to heels.

Keeping abs tight and hips level, use elbows to trace letters of your first and last name, allowing ball to move slightly from side to side (aim to write for about 30 to 40 seconds).

Do 4 reps.

Bikini Body Routine

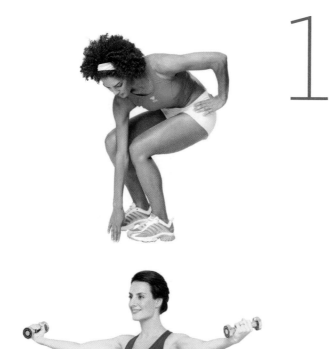

1 SINGLE-LEG SQUAT TOUCHDOWN

Targets abs, butt, quads, hamstrings

Stand with feet hip-width apart, knees slightly bent, hands on hip.

Lift right foot a few inches off floor. Squat, keeping left knee behind toes.

Then reach right hand toward left foot with back flat.

Slowly return to start.

Do 15 reps, keeping right foot lifted throughout; switch sides and repeat.

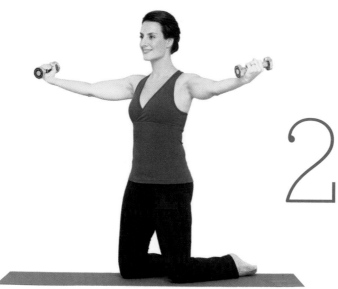

2 LOTUS

Targets back, shoulders, abs

Kneel upright on floor with knees under hips, back flat, shoulders down, abs engaged, holding a dumbbell in each hand, arms by sides.

Extend arms out to sides at shoulder level, palms facing up. Exhale and raise arms overhead.

Inhale and slowly lower arms back to shoulder level.

Do 10 reps.

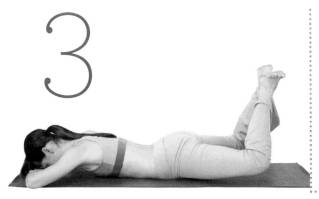

3

GRASSHOPPER
Targets butt, legs

Lie facedown on floor with elbows bent out to sides, forehead on top of hands, and lift extended legs a few inches off floor in V position, toes pointed out to sides.

Engage abs and press hips into floor. Keeping legs lifted, flex feet and bend knees, bringing legs toward butt. Tap heels together; release.

Do 10 reps, without touching legs to floor.

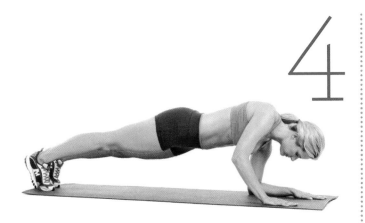

4

PLANK WALKUP
Targets arms, abs, chest, back, glutes

Get into plank position, balancing on floor on forearms and toes.

Keeping back straight, abs engaged and legs together, extend right arm, then left to press up into full push-up position.

Gently "walk" hands back down to plank, lowering onto right forearm, then left forearm.

Do 5 reps without lowering to floor.

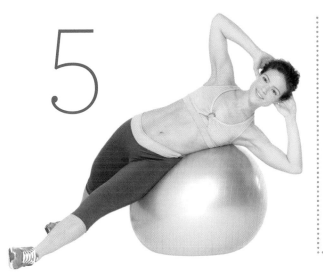

5

SIDE WALL CRUNCH
Targets abs, obliques

Place stability ball about 2 feet in front of wall. Lie faceup on ball with hips on its center, feet on floor about 3 feet apart, toes pointing to left and soles pressing against bottom of wall.

Put hands behind head, elbows out to sides, and rotate torso so that upper body faces left.

Keeping lower body still, crunch up while rotating torso to center; rotate back to left as you lower.

Do 15 reps; switch sides, toes pointing right and repeat.

WORKOUT 4

A Strong, Sleek Physique

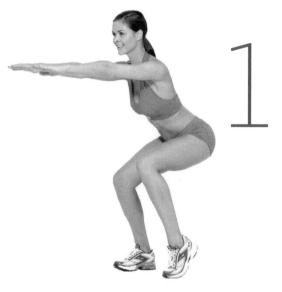

1

CALF RAISE SQUAT
Targets butt, quads, hamstrings

Stand with feet shoulder-width apart, knees slightly bent, arms extended at shoulder level in front of you, palms down.

Squat slowly, keeping knees behind toes and abs engaged, hinging forward slightly from hips.

Hold squat and lift left heel off floor (on tip-toes); lower and lift right heel off floor; lower. Squeeze glutes to stand back up.

Do 10 reps. Switch sides and repeat.

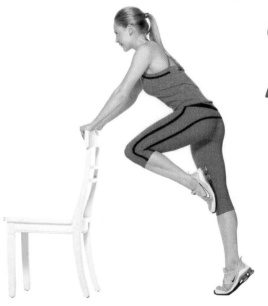

2

TREE TWIST
Targets hips, butt, calves

Stand a couple of feet behind chair, on tiptoes, with feet together, hands on top of chair back.

Keeping back flat, hinge forward slightly from waist and lift bent left knee to hip level in front of you, left foot by right knee.

Keeping upper body still and left foot by right knee, slowly bring left knee directly out to side; slowly return knee to center.

Do 10 reps, staying on tiptoes; switch legs and repeat.

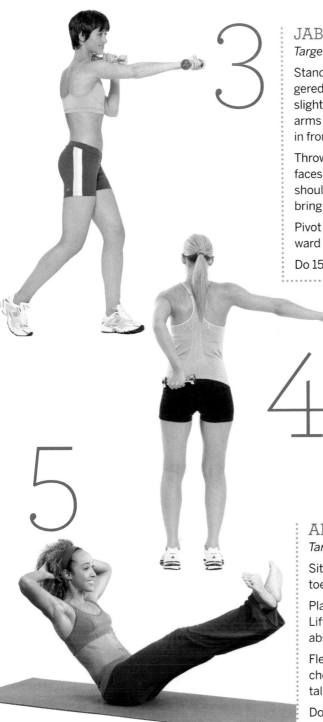

JAB, JAB, CROSS
Targets upper back, triceps, legs

Stand with feet shoulder-width apart and staggered (left foot forward, right foot back), knees slightly bent, holding a dumbbell in each hand, arms by sides. Bend elbows, bringing dumbbells in front of shoulders, palms facing in.

Throw a double jab: Twist thumb in so palm faces down as you punch left fist forward at shoulder level, then immediately bend elbow to bring dumbbell back in and repeat.

Pivot right foot to left and punch right fist forward at shoulder level.

Do 15 reps; switch sides and repeat.

BACK TOUCH
Targets back, shoulders, biceps

Holding a dumbbell in each hand, stand with feet hip-width apart, arms by sides. Extend arms diagonally out to sides so they're about one foot behind you, palms down.

Bend left elbow and touch back with dumbbell; extend. Switch arms and repeat to complete 1 rep.

Do 15 reps.

AERIAL PLIÉ
Targets abs, legs

Sit on floor with legs extended, heels together, toes pointed out to sides.

Place hands behind head, elbows out to sides. Lift legs about 2 feet, lean back 45 degrees, abs engaged.

Flex feet, heels together, and bend knees into chest (like a frog); extend legs, keeping back tall and heels together.

Do 15 reps.

Allover Toners

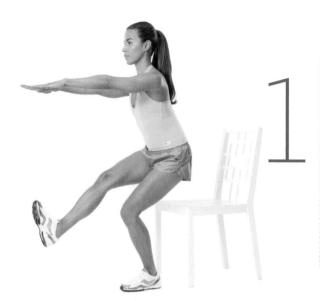

1

SEATED ONE-LEGGED SQUAT
Targets hips, butt, quads

Sit on chair with left foot on floor and right foot lifted about 12 inches, arms extended at shoulder level in front of you, palms down.

Pressing through left heel, lean body slightly forward and stand up, squeezing glutes.

Sit back down, keeping right foot lifted throughout.

Do 8 to 10 reps; switch legs and repeat.

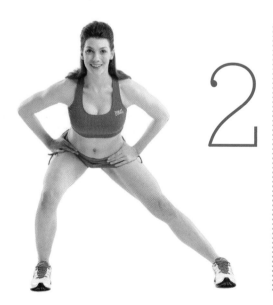

2

SIDE LUNGE JUMP
Targets butt, legs

Stand with feet hip-width apart, knees slightly bent, hands on hips.

Lunge right leg to right side, bending right knee 90 degrees and keeping left leg straight, hinging forward slightly from hips.

Step right leg back to start.

Do a half-squat, with knees slightly bent, then immediately jump straight up with both feet, bending elbows by sides so fists are in front of chest; land in half-squat.

Switch legs and repeat to complete 1 rep.

Do 10 reps.

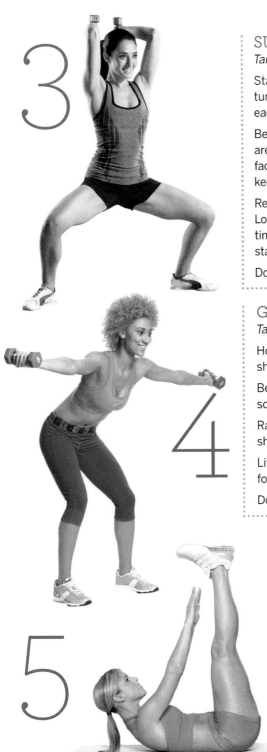

3

SUMO POWER
Targets triceps, butt, inner thighs

Stand with feet more than shoulder-width apart, toes turned out to sides 45 degrees, holding a dumbbell in each hand, arms by sides.

Bend elbows 90 degrees beside ears so that forearms are parallel to floor, dumbbells are behind head, palms facing each other. Maintaining arm position, squat, keeping knees behind toes.

Return to standing as you extend right arm overhead. Lower dumbbell behind head and repeat squat, this time extending left arm overhead as you return to standing, to complete 1 rep.

Do 10 reps.

GIMME A Y! GIMME A T!
Targets shoulders, upper back, abs, butt, legs

Holding a dumbbell in each hand, stand with feet shoulder-width apart, arms by sides, palms in.

Bend knees slightly, hinging forward slightly from hips, so back is nearly parallel to floor.

Raise arms up and diagonally overhead to form a Y shape, palms up. Lower arms by sides; do 8 to 10 reps.

Lift arms out to sides at shoulder level, palms up to form a T shape; lower arms by sides.

Do 8 to 10 reps.

4

PIKE AND EXTEND
Targets abs, legs

Lie faceup on floor with legs extended over hips, arms extended toward ceiling. Crunch up, reaching hands toward feet.

Keeping legs straight, lower arms back behind head as you lower upper back and left leg toward floor.

Crunch up, lifting left leg over hips and reaching hands to toes. Switch legs and repeat to complete 1 rep.

Do 10 reps.

5

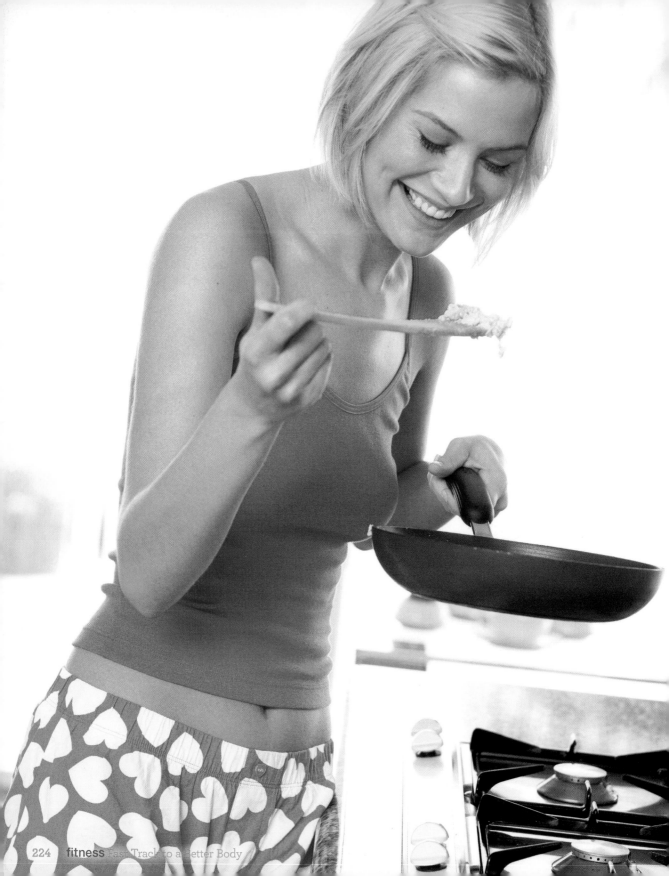

Foods for a Better Body

Get a head-to-toe boost when you add these colorful, nutrition-rich options to your diet.

The latest research shows that one of the best ways to lose weight and improve your health is to eat a host of colors. Trouble is, eight in 10 people in the United States don't consume enough of a variety of colorful fruits and vegetables, which means they face a nutrient deficit, according to a recent analysis of data from the National Health and Nutrition Examination Surveys and the USDA. Here's a kaleidoscope of inspiration to punch up your next meal.

Red

Burn calories. The new breakfast of champions is red chili peppers—seriously. People whose morning meal included the spicy vegetable were less hungry after breakfast and ate less fat at lunch, a study in the *British Journal of Nutrition* found.

Fresh idea: Add diced red chili peppers to scrambled eggs or top a whole-wheat English muffin with low-fat ricotta cheese and chopped chilies.

Step up your sweat session. Go longer by tossing beets into your salad. Scientists found that this vegetable helped cyclists increase their endurance by up to 16 percent. "Beets seem to reduce the amount of oxygen the body uses during exercise," says physiologist Stephen Bailey of Exeter University in England. "The result is muscles that can tolerate high-intensity exercise longer."

Fresh idea: Drizzle beets with red wine vinegar and olive oil, then roast. Or sauté with onions and garlic.

Orange

Outrun muscle cramps. Potassium has been shown to fend off mid-exercise cramping. If you want to up your intake, dig in to a sweet potato; one baked spud contains nearly 30 percent more of the nutrient than a banana. Bonus: The veggie is a great source of muscle-building copper, too.

Fresh idea: Don't fry sweet potatoes. This cooking method actually reduces the amount of potassium they contain. Instead, mash or bake them for a bigger dose.

Think like a genius. Pumpkins, and especially their seeds, pack a zinc punch. Scientists discovered that people who took a zinc supplement laced with other micronutrients performed better on memory, reasoning and hand-eye-coordination tests than those who took the micronutrients alone.

Fresh idea: Whip up pumpkin muffins or pumpkin pancakes. Toss some roasted seeds onto a salad for a flavorful crunch.

Yellow

See more clearly. Here's another reason to enjoy yellow corn on the cob tonight: It's packed with the antioxidants zeaxanthin and lutein, which work together to block harmful light that can cause damage to your eyes over time.

Fresh idea: Add frozen kernels to your favorite gazpacho recipe, or spread a mixture of butter, chopped fresh herbs (try basil and oregano) and a pinch of salt on corn on the cob.

Green

Slim down. Pears may help you kick hunger. Researchers in Brazil put two groups of overweight women on almost identical diets. The only difference was that one group ate about three small pears a day; the other had oat cookies with the same number of calories. The result: The fruit eaters lost more weight. Because pears contain water and are an excellent source of fiber, they keep you full longer. Plus, the fiber guards against drastic blood sugar spikes that can lead to overeating.

Fresh idea: Core pears, drizzle with honey, and bake for a sweet treat. Or add them to a grilled cheese sandwich.

Lift your mood. Feeling frazzled? Instead of reaching for a candy bar, try an avocado. It's packed with monounsaturated fat, which provides a pick-me-up.

Fresh idea: Drizzle sliced avocado with lime juice, brush with olive oil and grill; then season with salt. Or make kebabs with avocado chunks, grape tomatoes and mini mozzarella balls.

Purple

Fight the flu. Move over, chicken noodle soup. If you need to ward off sniffles, try plums. They contain neochlorogenic and chlorogenic acids, natural compounds that have been shown to inhibit the growth of viruses and bacteria in lab tests.

Fresh idea: Instead of jelly, put thinly sliced plum on a peanut butter sandwich. Or puree the fruit, pour it into ice cube trays and freeze it to use in summer drinks.

Fuel up for a workout. For a dose of energy, raisins are an excellent pre-workout snack. Athletes who ate the dried fruit 45 minutes before an hour of exercise performed just as well as those who had a sports gel, according to San Diego State University researchers.

Fresh idea: Pop a few raisins before or during a run for some additional get-up-and-go.

White

Build up your bones. Leeks are great for fending off osteoporosis because they're packed with inulin, a plant fiber that has been shown to increase calcium absorption by up to 33 percent. The key is to enjoy them with calcium-rich eats like legumes and dairy.

Fresh idea: Caramelize sliced leeks in olive oil or use 1 percent milk to make a chilled low-fat cream-of-leek soup.

Make It Happen!

We went straight to the people who (almost) never skip a workout to find out how they do it. Borrow their secrets and reach your goal, today.

Despite what you may think, the trick to exercising regularly isn't finding your inner enforcer. Rather, "it's getting creative and tapping your natural motivations," says Kelly McGonigal, Ph.D., a health psychologist and fitness instructor at Stanford. FITNESS asked women who work up a sweat almost every day for their stick-with-it solutions and picked these seven fail-proof favorites.

1. Don't put away your gear. From the moment she rises, Kristina Mone't Cox, 26, has exercise on the brain. That's because the first things she sees are her sneakers and workout clothes. "I've got them next to the bed in plain sight," says Kristina, the CEO of a communications firm in Houston. "I've also got dumbbells right where I can see them in the bathroom, and a balance ball, a yoga mat and a jump rope strategically placed throughout the house." Forgetting to exercise is never her problem.

Why it works: Visual cues act as a wake-up call. "We all have competing priorities like work, family, chores. Sometimes we need a reminder to keep exercise at the forefront," McGonigal says.

Do it yourself: If you don't have the space to display your gear (or if it'll mess with your decor), choose just one or two prime locations that you never miss. Better yet, "pick places where you spend a lot of time and can use the equipment, like by the TV or the phone," says Amanda Visek, Ph.D., assistant professor of sport and exercise psychology at George Washington University in Washington, D.C.

2. Turn your commute into a workout. On days that Monica Vazquez, 27, a master trainer for New York Sports Clubs in New York City, can't do her usual run, she stuffs her essentials—keys, cash, credit card, phone and ID—into a fanny pack and jogs home from work instead. "Running is a great workout, but it's also great transportation," she says. "Sometimes I get home even earlier than I normally do taking the subway."

Why it works: Running, walking or biking somewhere you have to go anyway makes exercise feel time-efficient. "And you don't have to carve out another part of your day for it," says Michelle Fortier, Ph.D., professor of health sciences at the University of Ottawa. "It's an effective strategy for people who are busy from morning to night."

Do it yourself: Your logistics may be a bit more complex if you drive to work or don't have good public transportation at your disposal. Maybe you can carpool in the morning or park your car a mile from the office and speed-walk the distance to and from your job. If you don't have a safe place at work to stash your stuff, invest in a lightweight backpack with waist and chest straps or swap your purse for a fanny pack on days that you plan to run home.

3. Invest in more workout clothes. For years, Gina Cancellaro, 36, a paralegal in Bronxville, New York, owned only one sports bra. "I didn't want to spend the money," she admits. Then one day she realized that this was a barrier to her working out: "My usual excuse was that it wasn't clean." So she loaded up on bras—and cute tops and shorts—at the mall. Now she exercises five days a week.

Why it works: "Having the right clothing doesn't just remove a hurdle; it reinforces your identity as an exerciser," McGonigal says. "And when exercising is an integral part of your identity, it isn't optional anymore. It's just part of your life." Plus, you've got to wear those adorable new workout clothes somewhere.

Do it yourself: Stock up on at least a week's worth of gym outfits to eliminate any last-minute handwashing in the sink. Think of it as spending now to save yourself grief later. To truly simplify your life, you may want to get several of the same tops and bottoms. "There's no time-consuming decision making that way," says Patricia Moreno, a FITNESS advisory board member and body and mind coach for the website SatiLife. "Look for basics that are comfy and show off your assets—whether that's your shoulders or your abs—so you feel good just suiting up."

4. Log your workouts online. A surprising thing happened when Michelle Busack, 38, started to post her exercise routines on Facebook: Old friends from high school whom she hadn't seen in years began writing comments. "At first they just congratulated me," says Michelle, a nurse in Columbus, Indiana. "But now we've bonded over this and they're my biggest cheerleaders." In fact, if she doesn't post a workout update for a few days, they'll demand to know what's going on.

Why it works: Social networking sites like Facebook and DailyMile offer an extra layer of social support. "You've got potentially all of your online contacts holding you accountable," says physiologist Michele Olson, Ph.D.

Do it yourself: Choose a social platform or online fitness tool (check out ours at www.fitnessmagazine.com/fitnesstracker). Then get in the habit of chronicling your progress after your workout every day so that your friends know when you usually exercise—and when you've slacked off. Post your minutes, your miles or whatever motivates you most.

5. Involve your causes. A political junkie, Rachel Simpson, 31, decided to use her partisan loyalties to help herself lose weight. She vowed to exercise four times a week; for each week she failed to do so, she agreed on Stickk (a website that helps people stay committed to their goals) to donate $25 to the library of a former president she didn't like. "Suddenly, working out was mandatory!" says the recent law school graduate in Minneapolis. Three months later she was down 16 pounds—and hadn't betrayed her party.

Why it works: Strong feelings, especially antipathies, have a multiplier effect. "Losing $10 to an enemy feels like $20 or even $30, so you push yourself harder," says Dean Karlan, Ph.D., professor of economics at Yale and a founder of Stickk.

Do it yourself: On Stickk, you can pledge to give a minimum of $5 to a charity or an individual (you provide the name and address) you like if you meet your goal or to one you dislike if you fall short. (Your credit card is charged.) Or sign up to raise money for a charity on the website Plus 3 Network: You pick from a list of goals that have prearranged corporate sponsors; if you meet yours, they'll pay the charity.

6. Make friends with class regulars. The thought of spending time with her Spinning buddies pushes Marie Bruce, 24, a coach and events director in Austin, Texas, to her morning class three times a week. "We're a tight-knit group," she says. "If I'm grumpy when I walk in, they don't let me stay that way for long." During the past six years, she's grown close to her extended gym family; in fact, they're invited to her upcoming wedding.

Why it works: It's smart time management. "You get your social fix while doing physical activity," Fortier says. Both boost health, and the better you feel, the likelier you are to want to exercise.

Do it yourself: Some classes foster friendships more than others, so you'll have to do some sleuthing. "Arrive early and observe," suggests Moreno, who teaches IntenSati, a mix of aerobics, dance, yoga and kickboxing. "Are people staking out their places in silence, or are they chatting and laughing and flitting around the room?" Another good sign: The instructor seems to know everyone's name.

7. Create an exercise contest. Taking a page from *The Biggest Loser,* Elizabeth Kirat, 35, and her friends are embroiled in a sweaty battle to see who can diet and exercise off the most weight. Every six weeks, they call the winner. "There's money at stake, but it's really the bragging rights that keep you returning to the treadmill," says Elizabeth, a photographer in Denville, New Jersey. So far she's dropped 10 pounds.

Why it works: Competition turns a solitary pursuit into a fun group one. "By trying to beat each other, you're actually pulling each other along," Visek says. "Even playful heckling validates that you're working toward a similar goal."

Do it yourself: The contest can be for anything: Most steps walked, most hours logged at the gym, highest percentage of body weight lost. Aim for anywhere from four to 10 participants. "Fewer than that, and one person who's not really trying can hobble the group. More than that, and it's hard for everyone to interact," Visek explains. To keep group members engaged, limit the competition to six-week rounds and have weekly check-ins, when people put money in the jar. "Your incentive is regularly refreshed in your mind that way," Visek says. Once everyone has agreed to the rules, let the games begin!

8. Go ahead, fill in the blank: _____
What will be your inspiration to give your body its slimming, sculpting, rejuvenating dose of exercise each week? Maybe, like the editors of FITNESS, you'll keep a secret stash of gym clothes in your desk drawer or wear a ponytail holder on your wrist as a reminder that a sleeker physique is just 15 minutes away. One thing is for sure: Consider this book your workout buddy, and the results you see will be all the motivation you need to get moving.

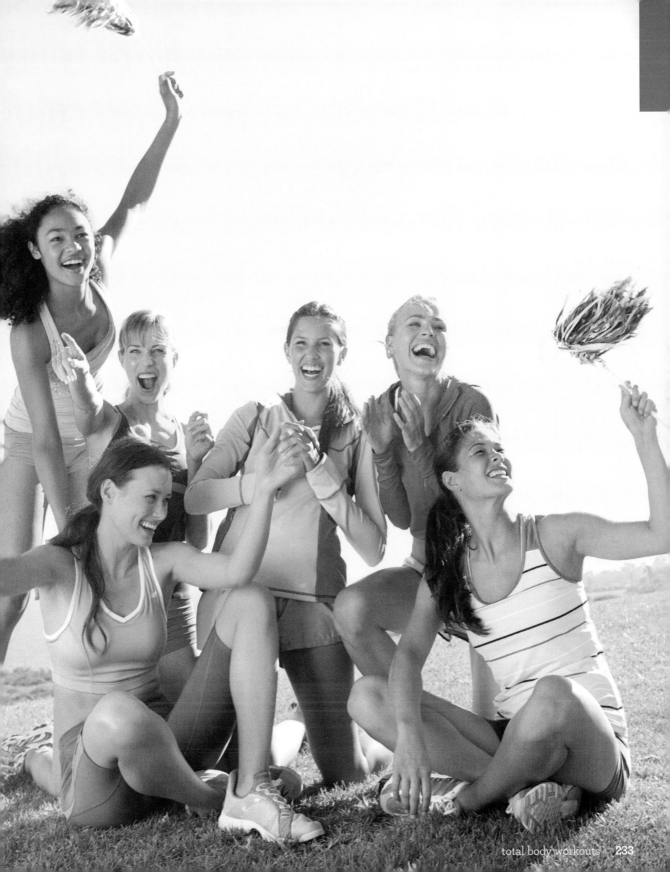

You Can Do It!

Endnote from the FITNESS editors

There's a reason the advice you read in FITNESS rings true: As editors, we don't just type it, we live it. From years of covering our beats, we've each picked up some tactics to stay motivated when energy is low, time is tight or that sugar fix is calling.

"I turn tough workouts into a game," says articles director Julia Savacool who is our resident mind-body pro. "Can I really do another three reps? Can I really survive another 800 meters at this pace? Reframing a slog as a fun challenge makes all the difference."

Others of us play a game of chicken. "I leave for work in a ponytail, no makeup, Lycra tights, with my office clothes in my bag," says deputy editor Mary Anderson, who oversees all exercise coverage. "This insures that I will stop at my gym and Spin if only so I can shower."

When it comes to sticking to a healthy diet, senior editor Bethany Gumper stacks the deck in her favor. "I fill the fridge with good-for-you foods so weeknight dinners are easy to pull together," says Bethany, who dishes up the latest science on weight loss.

And now we know why executive editor Pam O'Brien is impervious to the vending machine while juggling deadlines. "I bring a banana and an apple to work every day. The banana is my mid-morning snack, the apple is my afternoon snack," says Pam.

But perhaps beauty director Eleanor Langston best hit our main stay-fit inspiration. "I love feeling strong," says Eleanor. "It's so satisfying to finally do push-ups correctly, and being in shape makes me more focused in all areas of life."

We know this book will help you perform that perfect push-up, lose those last (or first) pounds—take your body to the next level. Here's a high-five for taking the first step.

index

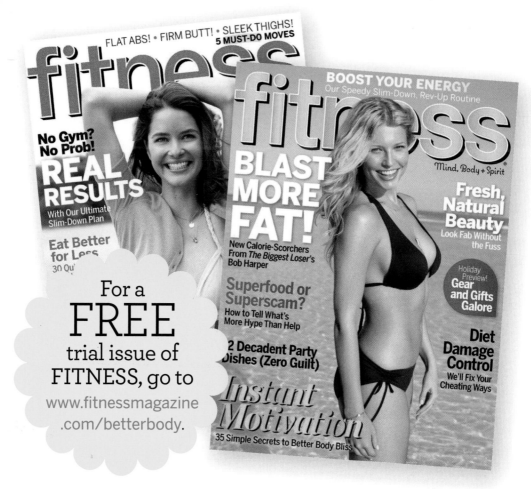

Trim and tone from head to toe

Boost your energy

Be happier and healthier

FITNESS MAGAZINE SHOWS YOU HOW TO DO
ALL THAT AND MUCH, MUCH MORE.